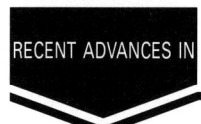

RECENT ADVANCES IN

Obstetrics and Gynaecology

RECENT ADVANCES IN OBSTETRICS AND GYNAECOLOGY

Contents of Number 18
Edited by John Bonnar

ISBN 0 443 04870 3

You can place your order by contacting your local medical bookseller or the Sales Promotion Department, Robert Stevenson House, 1-3 Baxter's Place, Leith Walk, Edinburgh EH1 3AF, UK
Tel: (0131) 556 2424; Telex: 727511 LONGMAN G; Fax (0131) 558 1278

Look out for *Recent Advances in Obstetrics and Gynaecology 20* in November 1996

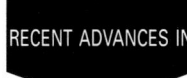

RECENT ADVANCES IN

Obstetrics and Gynaecology

Edited by

John Bonnar MA MD (Hons) FRCOG

Professor and Head, Department of Obstetrics and
Gynaecology, University of Dublin; Fellow of Trinity
College, Dublin; Consultant Obstetrician and
Gynaecologist, St James' Hospital
and Coombe Lying-in Hospital, Dublin, Ireland

NUMBER NINETEEN

CHURCHILL LIVINGSTONE
EDINBURGH LONDON MADRID MELBOURNE MILAN NEW YORK AND TOKYO 1995

CHURCHILL LIVINGSTONE
Medical Division of Pearson Professional Limited

Distributed in the United States of America by
Churchill Livingstone Inc., 650 Avenue of the Americas, New York,
N.Y. 10011, and by associated companies, branches and
representatives throughout the world.

Pearson Professional Limited 1995

First published 1995
ISBN 0443 052530
ISSN 0143 6848

British Library Cataloguing in Publication Data
A catalogue record for this book is available from the British Library

Library of Congress Cataloging in Publication Data
is available

The
publisher's
policy is to use
paper manufactured
from sustainable forests

Produced by Longman Singapore Publisher Pte Ltd
Printed in Singapore

Preface

Recent Advances in Obstetrics and Gynaecology 19 provides an up-date on many clinical topics which will be of particular interest to the practising obstetrician and gynaecologist. In recent years we have had numerous innovations in patient management which have not been subject to controlled trials. These require evaluation by well informed and experienced specialists. This issue contains a wealth of information from individuals who are recognised internationally for their expertise and knowledge in specific areas of patient care.

The Obstetric Section begins with a review of the advances in the treatment of ectopic pregnancy. Professor David Taylor and Dr A. N. Bhatt, from Liverpool, provide a detailed appraisal of the management of ectopic pregnancy by laparoscopic surgery. The results of the CLASP trial probably came as a surprise to many obstetricians. Mr Mark Kilby from Birmingham and Dr Keith Louden, from Bristol have had a special research interest into platelets and pre-eclampsia and they look at the role of low dose aspirin in modifying pre-eclampsia and fetal growth retardation. The diagnosis and management of fetal growth retardation are reviewed by Professor Martin Whittle, Birmingham, and Dr R. B. Beattie of Cardiff, and sound guidelines for patient care are provided. Dispute continues about the appropriate surveillance of the fetus in labour. This contentious area is carefully reviewed by Professor Peter Stone or Wellington, New Zealand, and Dr H. G. Murray, NSW, Australia. From Canada, Dr Jeff Ginsberg and Dr Joel Ray of McMaster University, Hamilton, examine the difficulties in diagnosis of thromboembolic disease in pregnancy, and provide new information and advice on management. The treatment of malignant disease in pregnant women requires a high degree of expertise to ensure the best results for the mother and at the same time minimising the risk to the fetus. Dr Des Carney, Medical Oncologist in Dublin, has wide experience in this area and he provides a comprehensive up-date for the obstetrician. The last chapter in the Obstetric Section is on audit in obstetrics by Dr Jean Chapple of London. I found this a fascinating and amusing chapter which shows the way forward and I would like it to be compulsory reading for all obstetricians.

The Gynaecology Section deals first with the subject of minimally invasive pelvic surgery. Dr Sean Duffy now heads the training unit for laparoscopic surgery at St James's University Hospital, Leeds, and he emphasizes safety and ways of avoiding the complications and mishaps which continue to occur and may result in litigation. New knowledge on polycystic ovarian syndrome is presented by Dr Frances Hayes and Dr Joseph McKenna, Clinical Endocrinologists with a major research involvement in this subject; useful guidelines on patient management are presented. Endometriosis continues as a major clinical problem and the cost of medical treatment has escalated. Professor Eric Thomas and Dr William Stones of Southampton have reviewed this area and they provide important data on cost effective management. For many gynaecologists bladder problems are an every day encounter and probably the most common are the unstable bladder and postoperative voiding dysfunction. Dr Gerry Jarvis of Leeds and Dr Timothy Sayer, Basingstoke, have particular interest in these problems and they provide excellent up-dates on the management of these bladder disorders. The management of faecal incontinence is now much more specialised and Mr E. S. Kiff and Dr James Hill of Manchester, provide important information for the gynaecologist on essential investigation and specific management. The volume concludes with a review of vulval dystrophy by Dr Noreen Gleeson who has recently returned to Dublin following her Fellowship in Oncology in Tampa, Florida.

I would like to thank all the contributors to the 19th issue for accepting the invitation to write for Recent Advances and adhering to the time schedule. I know that the readers will also be grateful to them for examining these particular areas and advising on the best and most up-to-date patient care.

I would like to thank Dr Gill Haddock and Churchill Livingstone for their assistance in ensuring the rapid publication of Recent Advances.

Dublin 1996   J.B.

Contributors

R.B. Beattie MD MB BCh BAO MRCOG
University Hospital of Wales Heath Park, Cardiff, South Glamorgan, Wales

Asit Narendra Bhatt MB BS MD MRCOG
Research Fellow, Department of Obstetrics and Gynaecology, Leicester Royal Infirmary Maternity Hospital, Leicester, UK

Desmond Carney MD PhD FRCPI
Consultant Medical Oncologist, Mater Hospital, Dublin, Ireland

Jean Chapple MB ChB FFPHM DROG DCH
Consultant in Perinatal Epidemiology, NHS Executive, London, UK

Sean Duffy MD FRCS MRCOG
Department of Obstetrics and Gynaecology, St James's University Hospital, Leeds, UK

Jeff Ginsberg MD FRCPC
Director, Thromboembolism Unit, Chedoke-McMaster Hospitals, Hamilton, Ontario, Canada

Noreen Gleeson MB ChB BAO MD MRCOG
Senior Registrar in Obstetrics and Gynaecology, Coombe Women's Hospital, Dublin, Ireland

Frances Hayes MB MRCPI
Research Registrar, Department of Endocrinology and Diabetes Mellitus, St Vincent's Hospital, Dublin, Ireland

James Hill FRCS
Consultant Surgeon, Hope Hospital, Stott's Lane, Salford, Manchester, UK

Gerry Jarvis MA (Oxon) FRCS FRCOG
Consultant Obstetrician & Gynaecologist, BUPA Hospital, Leeds, UK

E. S. Kiff FRCS
Consultant Surgeon, Withington Hospital, Manchester, UK

Mark Kilby MB BS MD MRCOG
Senior Registrar, Department of Obstetrics & Gynaecology,
Birmingham Maternity Hospital, Birmingham, UK

Keith Louden BMedSc BM BS MRCOG
Department of Obstetrics and Gynaecology, Southmead Hospital,
Bristol, UK

H. Murray BMedSc MB ChB MRCOG
Department of Obstetrics and Gynaecology, Westmead Hospital,
Westmead, NSW, Australia

Joseph McKenna MD FRCPI FRCP (Lond) FRCP (Ed) FACP ABIM
Department of Endocrinology and Diabetes Mellitus,
St. Vincent's Hospital, Dublin, Ireland

Joel Ray MD
Resident in Medicine, McMaster University, Hamilton, Ontario,
Canada

Timothy Sayer MD MRCOG
Consultant Obstetrician and Gynaecologist,
The North Hampshire Hospital, Basingstoke, UK

Peter Stone MB ChB MRCOG
Professor, Department of Obstetrics and Gynaecology,
Wellington School of Medicine, Wellington, New Zealand

William Stones MB BS DTM&H MRCOG
Lecturer, University Department of Obstetrics and Gynaecology,
The Princess Anne Hospital, Southampton, UK

David Taylor MD FRCOG
Consultant Obstetrician & Gynaecologist,
University of Leicester, Clinical Sciences Building,
Leicester Royal Infirmary, Leicester, UK

Eric Thomas MB BS MD MRCOG
Professor, Department of Obstetrics and Gynaecology,
The Princess Anne Hospital, Southampton, UK

Martin Whittle MD FRCP FRCOG
Professor, Department of Fetal Medicine, Birmingham Maternity
Hospital, Birmingham, UK

Contents

1

Advances in the treatment of ectopic pregnancy

A. N. Bhatt   D. J. Taylor

Recent evidence indicates that the incidence of ectopic pregnancy has been rising in some countries. In the USA, Goldner et al (1993) reported a fivefold increase in hospitalization for ectopic pregnancy, from 17 800 to 88 400 annually between 1970 through to 1989. In the UK the incidence of ectopic pregnancy has doubled in the decade 1980–90, and at present about 8000 ectopic pregnancies are treated each year (Department of Health 1994). In Leicestershire, England, 122 ectopic pregnancies and 9763 deliveries were recorded in 1993 giving a rate of 12.5 ectopic pregnancies per 1000 deliveries. In the City and Hackney Health District of London in 1990–91 the incidence of ectopic pregnancies was reported as 26.2 per 1000 deliveries (Irvine et al 1994). In France, Couturier et al (1994) reported 15 ectopic pregnancies per 1000 deliveries in Paris and the Provence-Alpes-Cote d'Azur during 1991–1992.

In the UK the direct maternal mortality caused by ectopic pregnancy decreased from 1.8 to 0.6 deaths per 1000 ectopic pregnancies between the trienniums 1976–78 and 1988–90. Ectopic pregnancy remains an important cause of direct maternal deaths accounting for 1 in 10 of all direct maternal deaths in the UK (Department of Health 1994).

Recently, with the development of immunoassays utilizing monoclonal antibodies to β-human chorionic gonadotropin (HCG) and high-resolution ultrasound scanners, an ectopic pregnancy can be diagnosed before significant haemorrhage occurs. This ability to make an early diagnosis coupled with the developments in endoscopic surgical equipment has led to new ways of treating ectopic pregnancy.

The treatment options are:

1. Surgical treatment: i.e. salpingectomy and salpingostomy through laparoscopy or laparotomy
2. Surgically Administered Medical (SAM) treatment i.e. administration of an abortificient into or around the ectopic pregnancy using endoscopic, radiological or sonographical techniques
3. Medical treatment: i.e. systemic administration of a cytotoxic agent

4. Expectant management: i.e. observation and monitoring until the ectopic pregnancy resolves.

SURGICAL TREATMENT

In 1884 Robert Lawson Tait described the operation of salpingectomy as a life-saving treatment for tubal pregnancy and for nearly 70 years this remained the treatment of choice for tubal pregnancy. In the English literature Stromme (1953) was the first to describe conservative surgery i.e. salpingostomy for tubal pregnancy. The first laparoscopic salpingectomy was described by Shapiro & Adler (1973) and since then the laparoscopic approach to surgical treatment has been developed and described with increasing frequency and improved outcome (Bruhat et al 1977; Bruhat et al 1980; DeCherney et al 1981). The current trend towards a more conservative and less invasive management of ectopic pregnancy is now feasible as a result of the developments in endoscopic instrumentation and techniques which have made surgical treatment relatively easy to perform (Young et al 1991).

Laparoscopic salpingectomy can be performed using laparoscopic scissors and diathermy (Alper et al 1992) or by using Endo-loop®. In the latter a loop of No. 1 catgut suture is first passed over the tubal pregnancy and then tightened. For safety and to prevent postoperative haemorrhage the pedicle should be secured with two loops of catgut. The tubal pregnancy is then cut distal to the loops and removed from the abdomen piecemeal or by using a tissue removal bag.

At a laparoscopic salpingostomy blood loss is reduced by first injecting the mesosalpinx with 10 to 40 iu of vasopressin diluted in 10 ml of 0.9% saline solution. The tube is then opened through an antimesenteric longitudinal incision over the ectopic pregnancy, using a fine diathermy knife (Lundorff 1992), a carbon dioxide laser (Paulson 1992), argon laser (Keckstein et al 1992) or simply by laparoscopic scissors, and ablating the bleeding points with bipolar diathermy. The ectopic pregnancy is evacuated by suction-irrigation ensuring haemostasis in the trophoblastic bed. It is important to remove only as much of the pregnancy as will come out easily, as enthusiastic removal of all tissue may provoke bleeding and require salpingectomy. The tubal incision is left open.

The two main areas of debate in the surgical treatment of ectopic pregnancy are: laparotomy versus laparoscopy, and salpingectomy versus salpingostomy.

Laparotomy versus laparoscopy

The question of whether the surgical treatment should be carried out through a laparotomy or through a laparoscopy has been addressed by prospective randomized studies. The major advantage of the laparoscopic approach over laparotomy is reduced duration of hospitalization and convalescence. Lundorff (1992) reported a reduction in the hospitalization time by 3 days, from 5 days to 2 days, in patients treated laparoscopically. In addition convalescence was reduced by nearly 2 weeks from 23 to 10 days. Similar results were reported by Nager et al (1992). Murphy et al (1992) reported no significant difference in the operative time between laparoscopy and laparotomy; however, patients treated through a laparoscopy had a significant reduction in estimated intraoperative blood loss, postoperative hospital stay, narcotic requirement, time to normal activity and total hospital cost. Lundorff (1992) carried out a second-look laparoscopy 3 months after the primary surgery and reported that the incidence of adhesions around the affected tube were significantly less in those treated laparoscopically, but the incidence of adhesion around the contralateral tube was no different.

Lundorff (1992) and Nager et al (1992) reported no significant difference in the incidence of persistent ectopic pregnancy. Seifer et al (1993) and Vermesh et al (1988) reported a 16% incidence of persistent ectopic pregnancy requiring further treatment after laparoscopic salpingostomy compared with 1% incidence after salpingostomy at laparotomy. The evidence to date suggests that the risk of further ectopic pregnancy and future fertility are not significantly different.

Maruri & Azziz (1993) examined the cost implications in the USA of using laparoscopy versus laparotomy in the treatment of ectopic pregnancy. They estimated that in 1987 at least 80% of ectopic pregnancies were suitable for laparoscopic treatment, representing 70 400 cases. If all the eligible patients were treated laparoscopically this would have resulted in a saving of approximately $138 920 000.00.

Salpingectomy versus salpingostomy

All tubal pregnancies can be treated by a partial or complete salpingectomy. However, in some patients salpingostomy may be more suitable. Salpingostomy is indicated where the patient wishes to conserve her fertility, is haemodynamically stable, the ectopic pregnancy is accessible and unruptured and not more than 5 cm in size, and especially when the contralateral tube is absent or damaged. In 167 patients with an absent or occluded contralateral fallopian tube, trying to conceive after salpingostomy for ectopic pregnancy, 91 (55%) patients had intrauterine pregnancy and 34 (20%) had subsequent repeat ectopic pregnancy (Thornton et al 1991).

In 1451 patients treated by salpingostomy for ectopic pregnancy either by laparoscopy or laparotomy, Kooi & Kock (1993) reported 759 (52.3%) intrauterine and 201 (14%) extrauterine pregnancies. These patients had both tubes present at the time of the salpingostomy. Dubuisson et al (1990) reported a 33.6% conception rate, 20% live birth rate and 12.8% repeat ectopic pregnancy rate in 125 women treated by salpingectomy for ectopic

Table 1.1   Therapeutic scoring system for ectopic pregnancy (EP)

Factors significantly affecting fertility after EP	Statistical weighting	Coefficient
Antecedent: one EP	0.434	2
For each further EP	0.261	1
Antecedent: laparascopic adhesiolysis[a]	0.258	1
Antecedent: tubal microsurgery	0.351	2
Solitary tube	0.472	2
Antecedent: salpingitis	0.242	1
Homolateral adhesions	0.207	1
Contralateral adhesions[b]	0.198	1

[a] Count only one occasion.
[b] If the contralateral tube is missing or obstructed, count as solitary tube.
Reproduced with permission from Chapron et al 1993.

pregnancy. Oelsner et al (1987) reported a 40.9% intrauterine pregnancy rate and 14.2% extrauterine pregnancy rate in 1630 patients treated by salpingectomy for ectopic pregnancy. Silva et al (1993), in a study of reproductive outcome after laparoscopic surgical treatment in 143 patients, reported overall intrauterine pregnancy rates for laparoscopic salpingostomy (60%) and laparoscopic salpingectomy (54%) as not significantly different. However, they found that a prior history of tubal damage was associated with a significantly reduced intrauterine pregnancy rate of 42% against 79% in women with no prior history of tubal damage. Ory et al (1993) concluded, from their retrospective cohort study of 88 cases of ectopic pregnancy treated surgically, that the choice of surgical treatment did not influence the post-treatment fertility and a prior history of infertility was associated with a marked reduction in fertility following the surgical treatment.

Chapron et al (1993) have described a scoring system, based on the patient's previous gynaecological history and the appearance of the pelvic organs at the laparoscopy, to determine whether the ectopic pregnancy should be treated by salpingostomy or salpingectomy. The rationale behind the scoring system is to decide the risk of recurrent ectopic pregnancy. If a patient is high risk for ectopic pregnancy then she would be better off having the tube removed and opting for *in vitro* fertilization and embryo transfer programme. Table 1.1 gives the therapeutic scoring system for ectopic pregnancy. Conservative treatment is advocated for scores 1 to 4, and radical treatment is advocated for scores 5 or more.

Persistent ectopic pregnancy (PEP)

This is a complication of salpingostomy and evacuation of ectopic pregnancy, when the removal of the pregnancy is incomplete and residual trophoblast continues to survive. The diagnosis is made by a lack of fall, or a rise in serum HCG level postoperatively. Untreated PEP can cause life-threatening haemorrhage and follow-up serum HCG estimation is essential in all patients treated conservatively.

PEP can be treated by a reoperation and further evacuation or salpingectomy. Recently, successful treatment of PEP has been reported with methotrexate given as a single intramuscular injection in the dose of 50 mg/m^2 body surface area (Hoppe et al 1994), or given orally (DiMarchi & Cyka 1992). Seifer et al (1994) reported treating 50 patients with PEP: 27 patients were successfully treated by salpingectomy; one of 16 patients treated with methotrexate, and one of 7 patients treated with salpingostomy required a third treatment in the form of salpingectomy; 32 patients out of 50 attempted conception and the cumulative clinical pregnancy rate after the treatment was 59% at 36 months.

SURGICALLY ADMINISTERED MEDICAL (SAM) TREATMENT

This technique requires the injection of a trophotoxic substance into the ectopic pregnancy or into the affected tube and has been carried out in a variety of ways. The aim of treatment is to obtain trophoblastic destruction without risk of systemic side effects. Several different substances have been tried with variable success rates i.e. from complete resolution of the pregnancy to failure. Table 1.2 lists the various SAM treatments used in the treatment of ectopic pregnancy.

Table 1.2 SAM treatment

Author & the year of publication	Number of patients	Agent	Access	Success n(%)	Tubal patency
Pansky et al 1989	37	MTX	Lap	33 (89)	19/21
Kooi and Kock 1990	25	MTX	Lap	24 (96)	
Kojima et al 1990	9	MTX	Lap	9 (100)	
Feichtinger et al 1989	9	MTX	TV	8 (78)	2/2
Menard et al 1990	17	MTX	TV	13 (76)	
Tulandi et al 1992	40	MTX	TV	28 (70)	
Fernandez et al 1993a	100	MTX	TV± IM	83 (83)	72/80
Risquez et al 1990	4	MTX	HSG	4 (100)	
Porreco 1992	3	MTX	TAb	3 (100)	
Goldenberg et al 1992	1	MTX	Hyst	1 (100)	
Vejtorp et al 1989	11	PGF$_{2\alpha}$	Lap	10 (91)	7/8
Egarter et al 1989	71	PGF$_{2\alpha}$+ Estrogen	Lap & IM	57 (81)	22/24
Lindblom et al 1987	27	PGF$_{2\alpha}$	Lap	24 (89)	
Lang et al 1990	15	PGF$_{2\alpha}$	Lap	13 (87)	5/6
Kiss et al 1993	1	PGF$_{2\alpha}$	Fallop	1 (100)	
Lang et al 1992	60	HyGlu	Lap	56 (93)	
Robertson et al 1987	3	KCl	TV	1 (33)	

MTX = Methotrexate
HyGlu = 50% Hyperosmolar glucose
KCl = 20% w/v Potassium chloride
Lap = Laparoscopy
Fallop = Falloposcopy
Hyst = Hysteroscopy

IM = Intramuscular injection
TV = Transvaginal sonographic control
TAb = Transabdominal percutaneous under sonographic control
HSG = Hysterosalpingographic control

Substances that have been injected into the fallopian tube or the ectopic pregnancy include: methotrexate (Pansky et al 1989), prostaglandin $F_{2\alpha}$ (Lindblom et al 1987), hyperosmolar glucose solution (Lang et al 1992), and potassium chloride (Robertson et al 1987). The local administration of these substances is carried out most commonly at laparoscopy, however, there are reports of this treatment carried out under ultrasonic control: transabdominal (Porreco 1992), transvaginal (Feichtinger et al 1989), radiological control (Risquez et al 1990), and falloposcopic control (Kiss et al 1993).

Lang et al (1990), in a randomized prospective trial, compared a local injection of hyperosmolar glucose solution with the combination of prostaglandin $F_{2\alpha}$ administered locally and systemically. They treated 16 cases with hyperosmolar glucose solution and 15 cases with local injection of prostaglandin $F_{2\alpha}$. All the patients treated with hyperosmolar glucose solution had complete resolution of the tubal pregnancy, whereas two patients treated with prostaglandin had an unsuccessful outcome. Tubal patency was confirmed by hysterosalpingography in seven of eight, and five of six patients from the respective groups. They reported three normal intrauterine pregnancies in the former group subsequent to the treatment.

Honigl et al (1993) have described no discernible effect of injection of hyperosmolar glucose solution on the histology of endosalpinx in a patient who had salpingectomy for incomplete tubal abortion 12 days after the injection. He has also reported a case of intrauterine pregnancy following a successful treatment of ectopic pregnancy in a patient with a single fallopian tube (Honigl & Lang 1992). Intrauterine pregnancy has also been reported in patients where ectopic pregnancy in their only remaining tube was treated by local injection of prostaglandin $F_{2\alpha}$ (Honigl et al 1992).

Porreco (1992) has described a technique of percutaneous, ultrasound-directed ablation of ectopic pregnancy with methotrexate. He reported success in the three patients treated. Risquez et al (1990) has described selective retrograde salpingography for diagnosis and treatment of tubal pregnancy. Under salpingographic control a specially designed catheter was advanced into the affected tube and between 5 and 35 mg of methotrexate was injected into the tubal lumen; in four patients surgery was avoided for the diagnosis and treatment of the tubal pregnancy. They claimed that the procedure was well tolerated and none of the patients had any side effects.

The success rate of ultrasonographic-directed local injection therapy is around 72% (Lindblom et al 1993). In laparoscopically treated patients where the pretreatment serum HCG is not more than 2500 iu/L, the success rate is more than 90% (Lang et al 1992). Transvaginal injection as described by Feichtinger & Kemeter (1989) would be suitable for use by gynaecologists skilled in oocyte recovery under ultrasound control.

Table 1.3 Medical treatment of ectopic pregnancy

Author & the year of publication	Number of patients	Agent(s)	Dosage regimen	Success n(%)	Tubal patency
Ichinoe et al 1987	23	MTX	0.4 mg/kg daily × 5 IM every other week	22 (96)	10/19
Sauer et al 1987	21	MTX+CV	1 mg/kg × 4 IM + 15 mg × 4 PO	20 (95)	15/20
Stovall et al 1991	100	MTX+CV	1 mg/kg × 4 IM + 15 mg × 4 PO	96 (96)	49/58
Prapas et al 1992	20	MTX+CV	1 mg/kg × 4 IM + 15 mg × 4 PO	19 (95)	17/20
Stovall & Ling 1993a	120	MTX	50 mg/m^2 IM	113 (94.2)	51/62
Bhatt et al 1994	16	MTX+CV	1 mg/kg × 4 IM + 15 mg × 4 PO	14 (87.5)	5/7
Bhatt et al 1994	19	MTX	50 mg/m^2 IM	16 (84.2)	

MTX = Methotrexate, CV = Citrovorum factor (folinic acid)
IM = Intramuscular injection, PO = Per oral.

MEDICAL TREATMENT

Methotrexate, an anti-folic acid metabolite, has been used successfully in the treatment of gestational trophoblastic diseases for nearly four decades. It has been also used to promote early resorption of placental tissues in abdominal ectopic pregnancy. The successful resolution of a tubal pregnancy with methotrexate was first described in 1982 by Tanaka et al. Since then there has been a growing interest in the medical treatment of ectopic pregnancy. Methotrexate has been the most commonly used drug by intravenous, intramuscular, and oral administration. Methotrexate interferes with synthesis of DNA by inhibiting synthesis of pyrimidines. This prevents the proliferation of trophoblastic cells leading to cell death. The trophoblast is then absorbed by autozymes and maternal tissues. The death of trophoblastic tissues in some cases leads to a tubal abortion of the pregnancy.

Over the years, several different regimens have been described with a success rate of almost 90%. Methotrexate has been used frequently with folinic acid rescue. Recently the use of methotrexate has been described as a single dose without the folinic acid rescue. Stovall & Ling (1993a) reported a prospective cohort study of 120 women with ectopic pregnancy ≤ 3.5 cm in greatest dimension, treated by a single intramuscular injection of methotrexate of 50 mg/m^2 body surface area, and 113 (94.2%) women had a successful resolution of ectopic pregnancy. The dose of methotrexate was repeated if the serum HCG failed to fall below 15% between day 4 and day 7. A repeat injection of methotrexate was required in 4 (3.3%) cases.

Post-treatment hysterosalpingograms demonstrated tubal patency on the ipsilateral side in 51 of 62 (82.3%) patients. Of those attempting pregnancy, 79.6% conceived with 87.2% being intrauterine and 12.8% being ectopic pregnancies. The mean time to achieve pregnancy was 3.2 ± 1.1 months. Table 1.3 describes some of the experience with systemic methotrexate in the treatment of ectopic pregnancy.

The main disadvantage of medical treatment with methotrexate is the incidence of side effects such as stomatitis, and elevation of liver enzymes. While these side effects can be easily controlled by early administration of folinic acid, their occurrence discouraged the use of systemic methotrexate. However, the single-dose regimen described by Stovall & Ling (1993a) is remarkably free of side effects even without the folinic acid rescue. The incidence of side effects is comparable to that following SAM treatment with methotrexate.

All patients treated with methotrexate need careful monitoring by regular clinical assessment, full blood count, and liver function tests to detect any side effects. Serum HCG levels should be closely monitored (at least once a week) until negative. Significant intraperitoneal haemorrhage has been known to occur after the serum level of HCG had fallen to less than 5% of initial pretreatment level (Bhatt 1994).

The medical treatment of ectopic pregnancy offers the advantages of minimal hospitalization, shorter time interval to normal activity, outpatient treatment, and better than 90% success in selected cases. When an ectopic pregnancy is diagnosed without laparoscopy (Stovall & Ling 1993b), medical treatment with methotrexate can eliminate the need for surgical intervention. Creinin & Washington (1993) compared the cost of surgical treatment and the methotrexate treatment for ectopic pregnancy, and concluded that the use of methotrexate substantially reduced cost and morbidity; the use of methotrexate in appropriate cases would have saved $280 million in 1991 in the USA.

The use of methotrexate in the treatment of persistent ectopic pregnancy following a laparoscopic salpingostomy is now well established (vide supra).

EXPECTANT MANAGEMENT

Before the advent of the salpingectomy in 1884, ectopic pregnancies were treated expectantly, carried a mortality rate of around 70% (Parry 1876) and the diagnosis was often made at post-mortem examination. Selected patients can now be managed expectantly and safely with a satisfactory outcome. Early diagnosis of ectopic pregnancy using high-resolution ultrasound scanners and serial serum HCG assays could potentially lead to the treatment of some ectopic pregnancies which in the past would have remained undiagnosed and resolved spontaneously. If the tubal pregnancies which are likely to resolve spontaneously can be identified then expectant management could be the treatment of choice. The problem lies in identifying the tubal pregnancies which are likely to resolve spontaneously. Work published from the Helsinki University Central Hospital may provide us with some clues to identifying such pregnancies.

Ylostalo et al (1993) have described selecting 127 (25%) out of 507 ectopic pregnancies over a period of 3 years for expectant management on the following criteria:

a. a falling level of serum HCG at 2-day intervals,
b. no sign of intrauterine pregnancy,
c. a diameter of the ectopic pregnancy of less than 4 cm, and
d. no signs of rupture or acute bleeding by transvaginal sonography.

The selected patients were counselled and instructed to contact the emergency unit if symptoms worsened. Each patient visited the outpatients department every 2 to 7 days for serum HCG estimations and vaginal sonography. Spontaneous resolution occurred in 72% of the selected cases (18% of all the ectopic pregnancies diagnosed). The other 36 patients (28%) were treated by laparoscopic salpingostomy, after an expectant management time of 2–18 days, for various indications such as pain, increasing volume of adnexal mass, increasing volume of fluid in the Pouch of Douglas or a constant or rising serum HCG level after the initial decrease. In one case tubal rupture occurred and was treated by laparoscopic salpingectomy.

Korhonen et al (1994) described the dynamics of serum HCG during spontaneous resolution of ectopic pregnancy. In 118 patients selected for expectant management, they described spontaneous resolution of 85% of ectopic pregnancies where the initial serum HCG was less than 2000 iu/L. In contrast, spontaneous resolution of ectopic pregnancy occurred in only 25% of cases where the initial serum HCG was more than 2000 iu/L. When the pregnancies resolved spontaneously, the serum HCG decreased to normal levels within 4 to 67 days (mean 20 days). Laparoscopy was indicated in two-thirds of the patients whose serum HCG levels remained at more than 64% of the initial level after 7 days. The percentage fall in the serum HCG by day 7 was found to be a better predictor of spontaneous resolution of ectopic pregnancy than the percentage fall of serum HCG by day 2. Interestingly half the patients in the study had initial serum HCG of less than 500 iu/L (below the detecting limits of some of the earlier pregnancy tests) and 73% of these had spontaneous resolution of the ectopic pregnancy. Atri et al (1993) reported a study of 13 patients (24% of all the ectopic pregnancies during the period) who were followed until spontaneous resolution of ectopic pregnancy. All these patients had initial serum HCG of less than 1000 iu/L and that decreased to normal levels within 3 to 45 days (mean 15.8 days).

Patients selected for expectant management must be properly counselled and followed until spontaneous resolution is complete. Tubal pregnancies have been known to rupture even when the serum HCG levels are low (Tulandi et al 1991). The expectant management of ectopic pregnancy should be regarded as experimental until we are able to predict successful spontaneous resolution with more than 90% accuracy.

UNCOMMON ECTOPIC PREGNANCIES

There are two groups of uncommon ectopic pregnancies: ectopic pregnancies at uncommon sites, and heterotopic ectopic pregnancies.

Cornual, interstitial, cervical, ovarian and abdominal pregnancies

While singleton tubal pregnancies account for 98.5% of all ectopic pregnancies, pregnancies at other sites create special problems and have been associated with greater morbidity and mortality than tubal pregnancies.

Cornual and interstitial pregnancies have been treated by laparoscopic surgical techniques with good outcome (Pasic & Wolfe 1990). Ovarian pregnancies have been treated by laparoscopic resection (Langebrekke & Bakke 1990), intramuscular injection of 50 mg/m^2 methotrexate (Shamma & Schwartz 1992), and local injection of prostaglandin $F_{2\alpha}$ (Koike et al 1990) into the gestational sac. Pregnancies in the rudimentary uterine horn have been successfully treated by local injection of methotrexate (Strohmer et al 1992). Cervical pregnancies, notorious for severe haemorrhage, were often treated by a hysterectomy and recently successful treatment with systemic methotrexate has been reported (Chao et al 1993), by transvaginal local injection of methotrexate (Timor-Tritsch et al 1994) and potassium chloride plus methotrexate (Marcovici et al 1994). Frates et al (1994) report successful treatment of four cases of cervical pregnancy by selective uterine artery embolization followed by dilatation and evacuation.

Heterotopic ectopic pregnancy

Another group of uncommon ectopic pregnancies is that of heterotopic ectopic pregnancies where at least one of a multiple pregnancy lies outside the uterus. The spontaneous occurrence of heterotopic ectopic pregnancy is rare: 1:30 000 to 1:2600 pregnancies (Richards et al 1982), but the incidence has been estimated to be as high as 1.2% in patients receiving *in vitro* fertilization and embryo transfer treatment (Dor et al 1991). Heterotopic pregnancy is a life-threatening condition and early diagnosis is extremely difficult. Serial HCG assays and ultrasonography are made unreliable by the presence of intrauterine pregnancy and mild ovarian hyperstimulation which is commonly present. The diagnosis is often made after the tubal pregnancy has ruptured. Even if diagnosed before significant intraperitoneal haemorrhage takes place, the choice of treatment is influenced by the presence of a viable wanted intrauterine pregnancy. Fernandez et al (1993b) have described six cases of heterotopic ectopic pregnancies treated non-surgically. Five of these cases were successfully treated without surgical intervention: three by injection of potassium chloride into the gestational sac and two by expectant management. Salpingectomy was required for one case 10 days into the expectant treatment.

In cases of heterotopic ectopic pregnancies where one of the pregnancies is in the uterus and viable, methotrexate and prostaglandins are contraindicated. In such situations injection of hyperosmolar glucose solution into the ectopic pregnancy may be the treatment of choice. Alternatively surgical removal of the ectopic pregnancy, with or without the affected tube, by laparoscopic or an open laparotomy approach should be carried out.

KEY POINTS FOR CLINICAL PRACTICE

1. While the incidence of ectopic pregnancy (EP) has been rising the maternal mortality caused by EP has been falling.

2. The trend is towards treating ectopic pregnancies more conservatively and less invasively.

3. Early diagnosis is the key to less invasive treatment for ectopic pregnancy.

4. With the developments in laparoscopic techniques most unruptured ectopic pregnancies could be treated without resort to laparotomy. Where available the surgical treatment should be carried out through a laparoscopy rather than a laparotomy because the laparoscopic approach reduces hospital stay, hastens patient recovery and saves on treatment cost. The future fertility of the patient is unaffected by the choice of access.

5. Surgically administered medical treatment can be used for ectopic pregnancy, with little risk of systemic side effects if suitable expertise and equipment are available. Methotrexate, hyperosmolar glucose, and prostaglandin $F_{2\alpha}$ have been used with 90% success in selected cases. These agents can be administered under laparoscopic, hysteroscopic, falloposcopic, sonographic, and hysterosalpingographic control. Patients must be monitored closely after the treatment until serum HCG is not detectable.

6. Systemic administration of methotrexate has been shown be an effective medical treatment of ectopic pregnancy. With the single-dose intramuscular methotrexate treatment regimen an ectopic pregnancy can be treated without subjecting the patient to any form of surgery. Since hospitalization is not essential in most cases, the medical treatment has been shown to be cheaper than the surgical treatment.

7. Up to 30% of all ectopic pregnancies may be suitable for expectant management, but at present these pregnancies cannot be identified.

8. While the newer treatment methods offer several benefits to patients and health care providers, patients with ectopic pregnancy should be properly counselled and carefully monitored. The patients should understand

the possible risks and have access to a 24-hour emergency unit in the hospital.

REFERENCES

Alper M M, Sperling A, Penzias A S 1992 Laparoscopic salpingectomy using conventional laparoscopy equipment. Int J Fertil 37: 26–28

Atri M, Bret P M, Tulandi T 1993 Spontaneous resolution of ectopic pregnancy: initial appearance and evolution at transvaginal US. Radiology 186: 83–86

Bhatt A 1994 Intramuscular methotrexate for tubal pregnancy: Failure and fertility. Am J Obstet Gynecol 170: 1840–1841

Bhatt A N, Anwar M, Taylor D J 1996 Intramuscular methotrexate in the treatment of ectopic pregnancy. (in press)

Bruhat M A, Manhes H, Choukroun J et al 1977 Essai de Traitment percoelioscopique de la grossesse extrauterine. A propos de 26 observations. Rev Fr Gynecol Obstet 72: 667–669

Bruhat M A, Manhes H, Mage G 1980 Treatment of ectopic pregnancy by means of laparoscopy. Fertil Steril 33: 411–415

Chao K H, Shyu M K, Juang G T et al 1993 Methotrexate treatment of cervical pregnancy: experience of four cases. J Formosan Med Assoc 92: 426–430

Chapron C, Pouly J L, Wattiez A et al 1993 Laparoscopic management of tubal ectopic pregnancy. Eur J Obstet Gynecol Reprod Biol 49: 73–79

Coutier E, Obadia Y, Rey D et al 1994 Rates of pregnancy outcomes in France. Br J Obstet Gynaecol 101: 155–156

Creinin M D, Washington A E 1993 Cost of ectopic pregnancy management: surgery versus methotrexate. Fertil Steril 60: 963–969

DeCherney A H, Romero R, Naftolin F 1981 Surgical management of unruptured ectopic pregnancy. Fertil Steril 35: 21–24

Department of Health 1994 Report on confidential enquiries into maternal death in the United Kingdom 1988-1990. Her Majesty's Stationery Office, London pp 61–67

DiMarchi J M, Cyka R E 1992 Oral methotrexate for persistent ectopic pregnancy. A case report. J Reprod Med 37: 659–660

Dor J, Seidman D S, Levran D et al 1991 The incidence of combined intrauterine and extrauterine pregnancy after in vitro fertilization and embryo transfer. Fertil Steril 55: 833–834

Dubuisson J B, Aubriot E X, Foulot H et al 1990 Reproductive outcome after laparoscopic salpingectomy for tubal pregnancy. Fertil Steril 53: 1004–1007

Egarter C, Fitz R, Spona J et al 1989 Behandlung der Eileiterschwangerschaft mit Prostagandinen: Eine meltizenterstudie. Geburtsch u. Frauenheilk. 49: 808–812

Feichtinger W, Kemeter P 1989 Treatment of unruptured ectopic pregnancy by needling of sac and injection of methotrexate or PGE_2 under transvaginal sonography control. Arch Gynecol Obstet 249: 85–89

Fernandez H, Benifla J L, Lelaidier C et al 1993a Methotrexate treatment of ectopic pregnancy: 100 cases treated by primary transvaginal injection under sonographic control. Fertil Steril 59: 773–777

Fernandez H, Lelaidier C, Doumerc S et al 1993b Nonsurgical treatment of heterotopic pregnancy: a report of six cases. Fertil Steril 60: 428–432

Frates M C, Benson C B, Doubilet P M et al 1994 Cervical ectopic pregnancy: results of conservative treatment. Radiology 191: 773–775

Goldenberg M, Bider D, Oelsner G et al 1992 Treatment of interstitial pregnancy with methotrexate via hysteroscopy. Fertil Steril 58: 1234–1236

Goldner T E, Lawson H W, Xia Z et al 1993 Surveillance for ectopic pregnancy – United States 1970 – 1989. MMWR CDC Surveillance summaries 42(SS-6): 73–85

Honigl W, Lang P F 1992 Intrauterine pregnancy in a patient with a sole remaining tube after local treatment of tubal pregnancy with hyperosmolar glucose. Fertil Steril 58: 625–626.

Honigl W, Lang P F, Weiss P A et al 1992 Intrauterine pregnancy after treatment of tubal pregnancy with local and systemic prostaglandins in a patient with a single oviduct. Hum Reprod 4: 573–574

Honigl W, Pickel H, Tamussino K et al 1993 Histopathology of the fallopian tube after local instillation of hyperosmolar glucose solution for unruptured tubal pregnancy. Fertil Steril 59: 1316–1318

Hoppe D E, Bekkar B E, Nager C W 1994 Single-dose systemic methotrexate for the treatment of persistent ectopic pregnancy after conservative surgery. Obstet Gynecol 83: 51–54

Ichinoe K, Wake N, Shinkai N et al 1987 Nonsurgical therapy to preserve oviduct function in patients with tubal pregnancies. Am J Obstet Gynecol 156: 484–487

Irvine L M, Hicks J L, Blair-Bell C et al 1994 The incidence of ectopic pregnancy in the City and Hackney Health District of London, 1990–91. J Obstet Gynecol 14: 29–34

Keckstein G, Keckstein S, Wolf A S et al 1992 Argon laser laparoscopy: an effective technique for conservative treatment of unruptured ectopic pregnancy. Int J Fertil 37: 82–85

Kiss H, Egarter C, Wnezl R et al 1993 Falloposcopic instillation of prostaglandin in tubal pregnancy. Lancet 342: 54

Koike H, Chuganji Y, Watanabe H et al 1990 Conservative treatment of ovarian pregnancy by local prostaglandin $F_{2\alpha}$ injection. Am J Obstet Gynecol 163: 696

Kojima E, Abe Y, Morita M et al 1990 The treatment of unruptured tubal pregnancy with intratubal methotrexate injection under laparoscopic control. Obstet Gynecol 75: 723–725

Kooi S, Kock H C L V 1990 Treatment of tubal pregnancy by local injection of methotrexate after adrenaline injection into the mesosalpinx: a report of 25 patients. Fertil Steril 54: 580–584

Kooi S, Kock H C L V 1993 Surgical treatment for tubal pregnancies. Surg Gynecol Obstet 176: 519–526

Korhonen J, Stenman U, Ylostalo P 1994 Serum human chorionic gonadotropin dynamics during spontaneous resolution of ectopic pregnancy. Fertil Steril 61: 632–636

Lang P F, Weiss P A, Mayer H O et al 1990 Conservative treatment of ectopic pregnancy with local injection of hyperosmolar glucose solution or prostaglandin $F_{2\alpha}$: a prospective randomised study. Lancet 336: 78–81

Lang P F, Tamussino K, Honigl W et al 1992 Treatment of tubal pregnancy by laparoscopic instillation of hyperosmolar glucose solution. Am J Obstet Gynecol 166: 1378–1381

Langebrekke A, Bakke T 1990 Laparoscopic treatment of ovarian pregnancy. Tidsskr Nor Laegeforen 110: 208

Lindblom B, Kallfelt B, Hahlin M et al 1987 Local prostaglandin $F_{2\alpha}$ injection for termination of ectopic pregnancy. Lancet i: 776–777

Lindblom B, Bengtsson G, Bryman I et al 1993 Medical treatment of ectopic pregnancy. Eur J Obstet Gynecol Reprod Biol 49: 80–82

Lundorff P 1992 Modern management of ectopic pregnancy. Early recognition, laparoscopic treatment and fertility prospects. Acta Obstet Gynecol Scand 71: 158–159

Marcovici I, Rosenzweig B A, Brill A I et al 1994 Cervical pregnancy: Case reports and a current literature review. Obstet Gynecol Surv 49: 49–55

Maruri F, Azziz R 1993 Laparoscopic surgery for ectopic pregnancies: technology assessment and public health implications. Fertil Steril 59: 487–498

Menard A, Hauuy J P, Crequat J et al 1990 Treatment of unruptured tubal pregnancy by local injection of methotrexate under transvaginal sonographic control. Fertil Steril 54: 47–50

Murphy A A, Kettel L M, Nager C W et al 1992 Operative laparoscopy versus laparotomy for the management of ectopic pregnancy: a prospective trial. Fertil Steril 57: 1180–1185

Nager C W, Wujek J J, Kettel L M et al 1992 Operative laparoscopy versus laparotomy for the management of ectopic pregnancy: a randomised prospective trial. The American Fertility Society 46th Annual Meeting

Oelsner G, Morad J, Carp H et al 1987 Reproductive performance following conservative microsurgical management of tubal pregnancy. Br J Obstet Gynecol 94: 1078–1084

Ory S J, Nnadi E, Herrmann R et al 1993 Fertility after ectopic pregnancy. Fertil Steril 60: 231–235

Pansky M, Bukovsky I, Golan A et al 1989 Tubal patency after local methotrexate injection for tubal pregnancy. Lancet ii: 967–968

Parry J S 1876 Extra-uterine pregnancy. Lea, Philadelphia

Pasic R, Wolfe W M 1990 Laparoscopic diagnosis and treatment of interstitial ectopic pregnancy. Am J Obstet Gynecol 163: 587–588

Paulson J D 1992 The use of carbon dioxide laser laparoscopy in the treatment of tubal ectopic pregnancies. Am J Obstet Gynecol 167: 382–385

Porreco R P 1992 Percutaneous, ultrasound directed ablation of ectopic pregnancy with methotrexate. A report of three cases. J Reprod Med 37: 363–364

Prapas J, Prapas N, Prapa S et al 1992 Conservative treatment of ectopic pregnancy with intramuscular administration of methotrexate (MTX/CV). Acta Eur Fertil 23: 25–28

Richards S R, Stempel L E, Carlton B D 1982 Heterotopic pregnancy: Reappraisal of incidence. Am J Obstet Gynecol 142: 928–930

Risquez F, Mathieson J, Pariente D et al 1990 Diagnosis and treatment of ectopic pregnancy by retrograde selective salpingography and intraluminal injection: work in progress. Hum Reprod 5: 759–762

Robertson D E, Smith W, Craft I 1987 Reduction of ectopic pregnancy by ultrasound methods. Lancet ii: 1524

Sauer M, Gorril M, Rodi K et al 1987 Nonsurgical management of unruptured ectopic pregnancy: an extended clinical trial. Fertil Steril 48: 752–755

Seifer D B, Gutmann J N, Grant W D et al 1993 Comparison of persistent ectopic pregnancy after laparoscopic salpingostomy versus salpingostomy at laparotomy for ectopic pregnancy. Obstet Gynecol 81: 378–382

Seifer D B, Silva P D, Grainger D A et al 1994 Reproductive potential after treatment for persistent ectopic pregnancy. Fertil Steril 62: 194–196

Shamma F N, Schwartz L B 1992 Primary ovarian pregnancy successfully treated with methotrexate. Am J Obstet Gynecol 167: 1307–1308

Shapiro H, Adler D 1973 Excision of an ectopic pregnancy through the laparoscope. Am J Obstet Gynecol 117: 290–291

Silva P D, Schaper A M, Rooney B 1993 Reproductive outcome after 143 laparoscopic procedures for ectopic pregnancy. Obstet Gynecol 81: 710–715

Stovall T G, Ling F W 1993a Single dose methotrexate: An expanded clinical trial. Am J Obstet Gynecol 168: 1759–1765

Stovall T G, Ling F W 1993b Ectopic pregnancy. Diagnostic and therapeutic algorithms minimizing surgical intervention. J Reprod Med 38: 807–812

Stovall T G, Ling F W, Gray L A et al 1991 Methotrexate treatment of unruptured ectopic pregnancy: A report of 100 cases. Obstet Gynecol 77: 749–753

Strohmer H, Boldizsar A, Feichtinger W 1992 'Chemical curettage' using intrauterine methotrexate injection. Hum Reprod 7: 1027–1028

Stromme W B 1953 Salpingostomy for tubal pregnancy: report of a successful case. Obstet Gynecol 1: 472–476

Tait R L 1884 Five cases of extra-uterine pregnancy operated on at time of rupture. Br Med J i: 1250

Tanaka T, Hayashi H, Kutsuzawa T et al 1982 Treatment of interstitial ectopic pregnancy with methotrexate: report of a successful case. Fertil Steril 37: 851–852

Thornton K L, Diamond M P, DeCherney A H 1991 Linear salpingostomy for ectopic pregnancy. Obstet Gynecol Cl N Am 18: 95–110

Timor-Tritsch I E, Monteagudo A, Mandeville E O et al 1994 Successful management of viable cervical pregnancy by local injection of methotrexate guided by transvaginal ultrasonography. Am J Obstet Gynecol 170: 737–739

Tulandi T, Hemmings R, Khalifa F 1991 Rupture of ectopic pregnancy in women with low and declining serum beta-human chorionic gonadotropin concentrations. Fertil Steril 56: 786–787

Tulandi T, Atri M, Bret P et al 1992 Transvaginal intratubal methotrexate treatment of ectopic pregnancy. Fertil Steril 58: 98–100

Vejtorp M, Vejerslev L O, Ruge S 1989 Local prostaglandin treatment of ectopic pregnancy. Hum Reprod 4: 464–467

Vermesh M, Silva P D, Sauer M V et al 1988 Persistent tubal ectopic pregnancy: Patterns of circulating beta human chorionic gonadotropin and progesterone, and management options. Fertil Steril 50: 584

Ylostalo P, Cacciatore B, Korhonen J et al 1993 Expectant management of ectopic pregnancy. Eur J Obstet Gynecol Reprod Biol 49: 83–84

Young P L, Saftlas A F, Atrash H K et al 1991 National trends in the management of tubal pregnancy, 1970–1987. Obstet Gynecol 78: 749–752

2

Low-dose aspirin: The rationale for preventing pre-eclampsia and intrauterine growth retardation: A role after CLASP?

K. A. Louden,   M. D. Kilby

Pregnancy-induced hypertension (PIH) is still a major cause of maternal mortality. In the last triennial report on Confidential Enquiries into Maternal Mortalities, 27 fatalities were directly attributable to hypertensive disease of pregnancy in the United Kingdom between 1987 and 1990 (DHSS 1994). This disease process, especially when complicated by proteinuria, is also responsible for considerable perinatal morbidity and mortality. In Nottingham (where both authors were Research Fellows), one-sixth of annual neonatal intensive care cots are attributable to babies born to women with hypertension. These two statistics exemplify the importance of maternal and perinatal morbidity and mortality associated with pre-eclampsia.

The pathogenesis of PIH is dependent, at least in part, upon the interaction between the surface endothelium in the uteroplacental circulation, the maternal platelets and the opposing action of eicosanoids produced by these tissues.

A method of protecting pregnant women from this disease process which affects 10% of primigravidae to a minor degree and 2% severely (Chesley 1978), would be of considerable benefit to mother and baby. Ideally, prophylaxis would be based upon an insight into pathogenesis, and would be simple, effective, inexpensive and have minimal side effects. Low-dose aspirin has the potential to satisfy these criteria, and over the last 10 years has been the focus of much obstetric and therapeutic interest. Scientific debate should not depend upon anecdote, but evidence from well designed prospective data collection. When such studies are small in numbers, then a meta-analysis may aid decision making as to the benefit of a therapy. The clinical experience provided by a meta-analysis of small and larger multicentre, prospective studies, including the *Collaborative Low-dose Aspirin Study in Pregnancy* (CLASP) (1994) have done much to answer whether low-dose aspirin is of use in the prevention of pre-eclampsia and to the drug's effectiveness and safety.

PATHOGENESIS OF PREGNANCY-INDUCED HYPERTENSION

Investigation into the pathophysiological mechanisms of PIH has been hindered over the years because of lack of a uniform definition for the disease process. The introduction of such a definition by the *International Society for the study of Hypertension in Pregnancy* (Davey and Mac-Gillivray 1986) should ensure that scientists and clinicians involved in research are at least comparing 'like with like'. The consensus of opinion seems to be that PIH affects predominantly primigravidae and is peculiar to pregnancy. The underlying pathophysiological changes seem to occur before the observed elevation in arterial blood pressure. The cardiac output in subjects with PIH is largely unchanged or reduced and thus the observed hypertension is thought to be secondary to an increase in total peripheral resistance (Groenendijk et al 1984). These haemodynamic observations are thought to be secondary to both increased tone in the arteriolar smooth muscle, via an increase in cytosolic free calcium (Kilby et al 1992) and changes in the microvasculature, especially the utero- and feto-placental circulations.

Vascular smooth muscle responsiveness to vasoactive substances, such as angiotensin II (A_{II}) is increased in individuals who already have developed PIH and prospective data have indicated that these changes precede any increase in arterial blood pressure, probably occuring in early pregnancy (Gant et al 1974; Baker et al 1991). There is evidence that this sensitivity may be secondary to an increased density of A_{II} receptors on arteriolar smooth muscle and mediated by a receptor-calcium coupling mechanism (Baker et al 1992). There is also evidence that this mechanism may be altered by endovascular thromboxane A_2/prostacyclin ratio, with a dominance towards thromboxane production.

Placental-bed biopsies have demonstrated that women with proteinuric PIH have an abnormality of placentation. The failure in the 'second wave' of endovascular trophoblastic invasion, a process that usually occurs between 14–18 weeks, leads to the formation of low-resistance vasculature within the uteroplacental circulation (Robertson et al 1967). This process leads to striking changes in both the micro- and macro-uteroplacental circulation and implicates this local circulation as being responsible, at least in part, for the increased peripheral resistance. In 'normal' pregnancy, the spiral arterioles are dilated, the musculo-elastic tissue in the vessel wall is replaced, and the endothelial cells are replaced by cytotrophoblasts. In pregnancy-induced hypertension, the changes are largely limited to the deciduo-myometrial junction leading to relative vasoconstriction between the radial and spiral arteries (Brosens et al 1972). These observed *in vitro* changes in the placental circulation may accurately relect *in vivo* events and could lead to a local sensitivity to vasoconstrictor stimuli and an alteration in the endothelial surface-mediated platelet activation (Roberts & Redman 1993). In proteinuric PIH (pre-eclampsia) there is *ex vivo* evidence of increased platelet activation (Ahmed et al 1991; Norris et al 1993) and exhaustion which seems to be dependent upon thromboxane A_2 production (Louden et al 1991).

EICOSANOIDS AND THE UTEROPLACENTAL CIRCULATION

Prostaglandins (PGs) are biologically active unsaturated lipids (C_{20} fatty acids with a cyclopentane ring) which are probably synthesized by all cells in the human body and have widespread biological actions. They are essentially *local* hormones acting at or near to their site of production and are inactivated in the pulmonary circulation (Bergstrom et al 1968). The major pathways of PG biosynthesis are shown in Fig. 2.1. There are two main types of prostaglandins, those synthesized from arachidonic acid (AA), *2-series*; and those derived from dihomogammalinoleic acid (DGLA), *1-series*.

Glycerolphospholipids derived from plasmalemmae are the most important source of AA and its liberation depends upon the activity of phospholipase A_2. Dihommogammalinoleic and arachidonic acids circulate as their esters and may be metabolized by the two microsomal enzymes, *lipo-oxygenase* and *cyclo-oxygenase* respectively, to form leukotrienes and prostaglandins. It is the effect of cyclo-oxygenase on AA which is probably the rate limiting step in eicosanoid biosynthesis.

It would be expected that the non-endothelialized vessels in the placental bed of 'normal' pregnant women would be susceptible to provoking platelet activation and aggregation (Wallenburg et al 1983), but this rarely seems to occur. This state of affairs is at least in part due to a relative excess in local production of prostacyclin (PGI_2) by the fetoplacental circulation (Myatt & Elder 1977). In vascular tissue, once cyclo-oxygenase has formed intermediate, unstable eicosanoids (PGH_2) from arachidonic acid, these are converted to PGI_2 (Moncada et al 1976). Prostacyclin is a highly unstable molecule that inhibits platelet reactivity and has a vasodilatory action (Moncada & Vane 1979). Its mode of action is mediated by increasing the intraplatelet cyclic adenine monophosphate concentrations (Tateson et al 1977).

Human blood platelets are anuclear, cytoplasmic fragments derived from megakaryocytes, that circulate as part of the cellular constituents of blood. These cells have the ability to undergo rapid response to physiologically occurring molecules released during endothelial damage. The 'activated' platelets aggregate onto endothelial surfaces and undergo exocytosis, releasing pro-aggregatory and vasoactive substances into the microcirculation. The physiology of the platelet is thought to be controlled by intracellular second messenger systems, which are modified in normal and pathological pregnancies (Kilby et al 1992). In platelets, the major eicosanoid produced is thromboxane A_2 (TXA_2) that is generated during surface mediated platelet aggregation and exocytosis. This prostaglandin has a short half-life of less than 30 seconds and in turn acts as an amplification system promoting further platelet aggregation and local vasoconstriction (Piper & Vane 1969). Thromboxane A_2 is non-enzymatically hydrolysed to TXB_2.

In normal pregnancy PGI_2 may protect the uteroplacental circulation from platelet deposition and have a local vasodilatory effect. The utero- and feto-placental vascular resistance seem to be dependent upon the balance between vasoconstrictors (i.e. A_{II}, endothelin-1 and TXA_2) and vasodilators (PGI_2 and nitric oxide). In pregnancy the synthesis of both PGI_2 (Lewis et al 1980) and TXA_2 (Greer et al 1985) by the feto-placental

Arachidonic acid metabolism

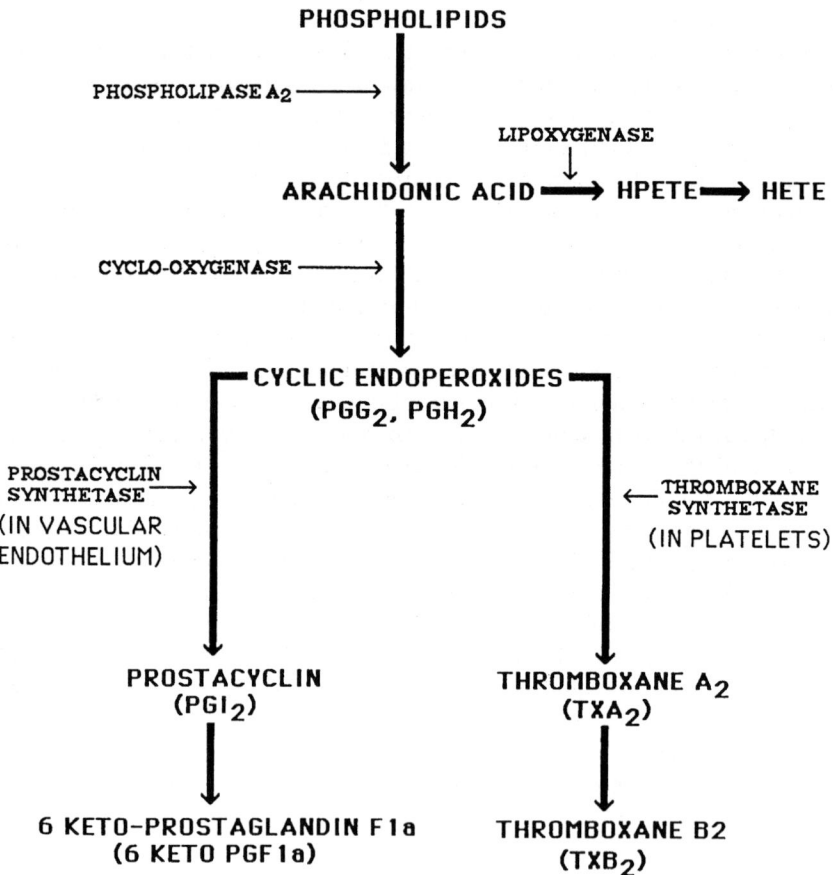

PHOSPHOLIPIDS

PHOSPHOLIPASE A2 ⟶

LIPOXYGENASE

ARACHIDONIC ACID ⟶ HPETE ⟶ HETE

CYCLO-OXYGENASE ⟶

CYCLIC ENDOPEROXIDES
(PGG_2, PGH_2)

PROSTACYCLIN
SYNTHETASE ⟶
(IN VASCULAR
ENDOTHELIUM)

⟵ THROMBOXANE
SYNTHETASE
(IN PLATELETS)

PROSTACYCLIN
(PGI_2)

THROMBOXANE A_2
(TXA_2)

6 KETO-PROSTAGLANDIN F1a
(6 KETO PGF1a)

THROMBOXANE B2
(TXB_2)

Fig. 2.1   The metabolism of prostaglandin formation in human pregnancy.

unit seems to be increased. However, the lack of a 'gold standard' assay to measure eicosanoids and their metabolites and the fact that metabolic pathways for such substances have not been fully delineated in either normal or abnormal pregnancies make interpretation of such findings difficult.

THE IMBALANCE BETWEEN PROSTAGLANDINS IN PREGNANCY-INDUCED HYPERTENSION

Many of the features of pre-eclampsia could be explained by a relative deficiency of PGI_2, and that this precedes the onset of overt disease (Fitzgerald et al 1987). Prostacyclin production by the feto-placental unit has been demonstrated to be reduced in PIH as compared with normotensive pregnancy of comparable gestation (Remuzzi et al 1980). Kinetic analysis of prostaglandin synthetase in umbilical artery microsomes showed a reduction in activity in pre-eclampsia (Downing et al 1982). However, these changes do not seem to be specific to PIH, as others have demonstrated similar data from pregnancies complicated by intrauterine growth retardation, (IUGR) (Stuart et al 1981). These two conditions may share a common aetiology in the failure of placentation (Khong et al 1986).

Several studies have reported an increase in TXB_2 and a decrease in PGI_2 metabolites in venous blood of pre-eclamptic counterparts. Perhaps the strongest of these studies is the prospective study carried out by Greer and colleagues (1985), in which TXB_2 and the stable metabolite of PGI_2, 6-keto PGF_{1a}, were measured by radioimmunoassay. In the pre-eclamptic subjects, a significant rise in TXB_2 was noted in the third trimester, while in normotensive counterparts the concentration fell. Conversely, the 6-keto PGF_{1a} concentrations were unrecordable in subjects who developed pre-eclampsia, but were comparable with normotensive groups at the beginning of the third trimester. Similar findings have been noted when measuring the urinary metabolites of prostacyclin (Fitzgerald et al 1987).

Another approach is the analysis of *in vitro* experiments. Such experiments are typified by those described by Walsh and his colleagues (1985) who used a homogenate of incubated placental tissue with subsequent radioimmunoassay of the incubation media and measurements of metabolites of TXA_2 and PGI_2. Obviously, extrapolation to the *in vivo* situation should be made with care, but a 50% decrease in PGF_{1a} production has been described (Walsh et al 1985) adding some credence to the 'imbalance' hypothesis.

The evidence, mainly from *in vitro* experiments, suggests that pre-eclampsia is a condition of relative prostacyclin deficiency, particularly within the placental circulations. This would increase platelet-endothelial interaction within the utero-placental circulation and predispose to spiral artery micro-thrombosis decreasing uteroplacental bloodflow. This alteration in eicosanoid balance may also contribute to the increased tension in vascular smooth muscle and loss of refractoriness to A_{II} that precedes the clinical syndrome of pre-eclampsia.

ASPIRIN: A ROLE IN PHARMACOLOGICAL PROPHYLAXIS FOR PREGNANCY-INDUCED HYPERTENSION?

The rationale for the use of aspirin is to reduce TXA_2 production and render platelets less aggregable, whilst maintaining PGI_2 production. Aspirin is a non-steroidal, anti-inflammatory drug which is derived from the bark of the Willow tree. In the past, obstetricians have discouraged generations of pregnant women from taking aspirin and other non-steroidal anti-inflammatory drugs as analgesics, because of fears of both maternal and fetal haemorrhage, and premature closure of the ductus arteriosus. Aspirin inhibits the enzyme *cyclo-oxygenase* which decreases the production of eicosanoids by cells. This effect may be used to influence prostacyclin/thromboxane production in the uteroplacental circulation (i.e. prophylaxis in pre-eclampsia and lupus anticoagulant) and in altering platelet function (anti-thrombotic effect).

Pharmacology of anti-platelet agents

Aspirin irreversibly acetylates the active site of the cyclo-oxygenase enzyme (Roth & Majeus 1975), which results in the decreased production of prostaglandins (the aspirin effect). Aspirin is de-acetylated to salicylic acid, which is also active in that it inhibits the conversion of hydroxy-eicosapentanoic acid by lipo-oxygenase. Thus, salicylate may increase platelet adhesion by affecting eicosanoid biosynthesis, which has a significant effect on platelet aggregation (the salicylate effect). These two effects are different and both aspirin and salicylate occupy different receptor sites. Their receptors are quite close together and thus these molecules may effect each others occupancy by 'steric hinderance' (de Swiet & Fryer 1990).

Aspirin is mainly absorbed through the small intestine, as a result of the dissociation of this molecule in the relative alkaline micro-environment. After aspirin absorption it is metabolized by hydrolysis in the gut (by plasma esterases) and in the liver. Hepatic de-esterification accounts for the major route of aspirin metabolism and this is variable between individuals (de Swiet & Fryer 1990). The concept of 'low-dose' aspirin is that cyclo-oxygenase is fully acetylated in the platelets of the pre-systemic (pre-hepatic) circulation, but insufficent aspirin is present in the systemic circulation to inhibit eicosanoid metabolism in other tissues, in particular the placental vasculature and the fetus.

In vivo studies in rats have shown that intra-duodenal aspirin spares systemic vascular prostacyclin (6-keto-PGF_{1a} production in aortic tissue), whereas intravenous aspirin caused a marked inhibitory effect on prostacyclin production (Benigini et al 1989). The first pass effect seems to protect the vascular endothelium against the effects of aspirin. A cross-over trial using both oral and intravenous routes has compared the effects on urinary thromboxane and prostacyclin measurements of relatively high-dose (1 g) aspirin in humans (Bucchi et al 1986). These data demonstrated that eicosanoid metabolites were not affected by oral aspirin, but were inhibited following parenteral administration. A further study, supporting these data, utilized coincident treatment with unlabelled oral and radio-labelled intravenous aspirin. Plasma drug concentration-time curves were compared to allow estimation of systemic bioavailablility. This ranged from 46% to 52% for doses of aspirin between 20 mg and 1300 mg, and were unchanged by chronic administration (Pederson & FitzGerald 1984). This indicates that the enzyme systems responsible for metabolizing aspirin were not saturated within the dose range studied. Serum thromboxane production was significantly reduced before any aspirin was detectable in the systemic circulation using mass spectrometry. This fact, combined with the finding that simulated peak plasma aspirin concentrations underestimate the inhibition of TXB_2 production after 20–40 mg of aspirin, are strong evidence for the pre-systemic acetylation of platelet cyclo-oxygenase using low-dose aspirin.

Ex vivo evidence for the use of low-dose aspirin in inhibiting platelet reactivity

Platelet aggregation is irreversibly inhibited by aspirin (O'Brien 1968), even at quite small doses (Nuotto et al 1984). Studies of platelet aggregation have been reported in various groups of patients who have taken 60 mg aspirin daily (Louden et al 1992). These studies have employed a 'whole blood' medium, which is more physiological than conventional 'platelet-rich plasma' since platelets are studied in their natural milieu along with red and white blood cells (Fox et al 1982). In addition to platelet aggregation, the release reaction of platelet storage granules, which can occur when platelets are activated, was also measured, along with platelet production of TXB_2.

In non-pregnant women, who received 60 mg aspirin daily for 10 days, there was a significant reduction in platelet aggregation and release reaction after *ex vivo* stimulation with both arachidonic acid (the precursor of TXA_2 via cyclo-oxygenase) and collagen (which acts partially via the cyclo-oxygenase pathway).

Eighteen normal pregnant women and 16 women admitted to hospital with PIH were randomized to receive either 60 mg aspirin daily or matched placebo. Cord bloods were taken at delivery to study the effect of maternal aspirin on the neonate (Louden et al 1990a). Platelet aggregation and release reaction after stimulation with arachidonic acid, collagen and adrenaline were all inhibited by treatment with 60 mg aspirin daily, in both the normal and hypertensive women. Interestingly, adrenaline-induced platelet reactivity is increased in normal pregnancy (Louden et al 1990b), and only then appears to recruit the cyclo-oxygenase pathway, hence becoming aspirin-sensitive. This observed increase in adrenaline-induced platelet reactivity in normal pregnancy with gestation is not citrate-dependent (Fox et al 1994). In proteinuric PIH, adrenaline-induced platelet reactivity was decreased (and hence the capacity for aspirin inhibition diminished), perhaps reflecting a failure to adapt to normal pregnancy, but more probably reflecting platelet exhaustion after activation and degranulation (Louden et al 1991; Louden et al 1992). Serum TXB_2 production was significantly reduced in all of the groups of patient who received 60 mg aspirin daily. Similar inhibition has been described when blood samples from pregnant women have been treated with aspirin (final concentration 100 µM) *in vitro* (Norris et al 1994). In studies using platelet-rich plasma instead of whole blood techniques, subjects treated with low-dose aspirin (and who had already shown evidence of platelet 'exhaustion' (Sullivan et al 1993)) showed increased platelet aggregation, suggesting that aspirin decreases *in vivo* platelet activation and reduces platelet exhaustion seen *ex vivo*.

Perhaps surprisingly, there were no statistically significant differences in platelet aggregation, the release reaction or serum TXB_2 production when the neonates exposed to maternal aspirin were compared with those who had been exposed to maternal placebo (Louden et al 1994). As the number of observations was small, there is the possibility of a type II error here, but the apparent relative sparing of neonatal platelet function is in marked contrast to the profound and comprehensive inhibition seen in the adults. The pre-systemic acetylation of maternal platelet cyclo-oxygenase with low-dose aspirin, as previously described, explains the inhibitory effect which was observed. However, it appears that at low doses, there is sufficient metabolism of aspirin in the pre-systemic circulation such that very little aspirin ever reaches the fetus.

Low-dose aspirin and the prevention of pregnancy-induced hypertension (observational and small prospective studies)

The first case report of the use of aspirin for the prevention of PIH involved treatment with '600 mg three-times daily' in a woman who had suffered recurrent severe pre-eclampsia in previous pregnancies (Goodlin 1978). At 32 weeks, successful delivery was accomplished as the blood pressure began to rise. Only after publication of this report did the patient confess to having only taken 85 mg daily, contrary to instructions (R. Goodlin, personal communication)! Using this low dose prospectively, treatment of a further five patients with early onset PIH resulted in an improvement in maternal symptoms and platelet counts, but without demonstrable benefit to the fetus (Goodlin 1983). Moreover, a retrospective questionnaire had shown that in 146 primigravidae, those who admitted to having taken aspirin at least once per fortnight during the pregnancy, were significantly less likely to have developed PIH than those who had abstained (Crandon & Isherwood 1979).

The first prospective randomized study to address this subject recruited 102 women (largely multigravidae) on the basis of a poor past obstetric history of pre-eclampsia or IUGR, along with other risk factors, and compared daily treatment with 150 mg aspirin and 300 mg dipyridamole, versus no treatment (Beaufils et al 1985). This combined anti-platelet regimen resulted in a greatly reduced incidence of pre-eclampsia (0% versus 13%) and major fetal complications (0% versus 20%). This study has been criticized, however, because of the heterogeneity of the groups studied, the lack of placebo control, and the use of two anti-platelet agents simultaneously. There is no objective evidence to suggest that the addition of dipyridamole adds to the clinical effectiveness of low-dose aspirin in pregnancy.

There followed a more rigorously conducted study which involved primigravidae who were deemed to be at risk of PIH on the basis of increased vascular sensitivity to an angiotensin II infusion at 28 weeks gestation (Wallenburg et al 1986). This study, in epidemiological terms, is small, but remarkable in a number of ways. In order to study primigravidae, and hence the population with the most important risk factor for the condition, 207 time-consuming angiotensin II infusions were required to yield a study population of 46 women deemed to be at high risk for the development of PIH. This uncompromising attitude to patient selection adds greatly to the significance of the results. The 46 women were randomized in double-blind fashion to receive either 60 mg aspirin or placebo, daily until delivery, and treatment resulted in a major reduction in the incidence of severe PIH and pre-eclampsia (0% versus 43%) and IUGR (0% versus 13%). This predictive test was performed at 28 weeks gestation, yet the first known pathological feature of PIH, the failure of the second-wave invasion of trophoblast, occurs much earlier in pregnancy. Thus, the apparently improved outcome in the aspirin group probably represents palliation of an existing disease process which has yet to manifest clinically, rather than true prevention.

Subsequent studies have continued to be hampered by the difficulty in selecting a group of patients, particularly primigravidae, who are genuinely at risk of pre-eclampsia. Concerns about any potential unwanted effects of low-dose aspirin (premature closure of ductus arteriosus, Reyes syndrome, bleeding tendency, etc.) have engendered an understandable reluctance to study a large population of normal primigravidae. Consequently, extrapolation of the results of the following studies into clinical practice is quite difficult, as specially selected patients have been recruited.

The roll-over test, in which the pressor response to a change in position from the left lateral to the supine is measured, was initially described as a predictive test for the development of PIH (Gant et al 1974). Performed at

28 weeks, those patients who exhibited a rise in diastolic blood pressure of 20 mmHg after rolling-over were found to be at risk of PIH. Although the failure of this test to provide consistent or clinically useful results has recently been highlighted (Wallenburg 1989), it was used as a screening test in a study of 791 women who where primigravid, had a previous history of 'pre-eclamptic toxaemia', or had a twin pregnancy (Schiff et al 1989). Sixty five women with positive tests were randomised to receive either 100 mg aspirin or matched placebo, daily until 10 days before the expected date of delivery. The subsequent development of both PIH (12% versus 36%) and pre-eclampsia (3% versus 23%) were substantially reduced in the aspirin group. The same group have subsequently published a small randomized placebo-controlled study of the effect of 100 mg aspirin daily on established mild PIH in primigravidae between 30–36 weeks, and found no clinical benefit (Schiff et al 1990).

Doppler ultrasound velocimetry has been used to select a group of patients who might benefit from low-dose aspirin. One hundred normal primigravidae who had repeatedly abnormal Doppler ultrasound velocimetry studies of the uteroplacental circulation at 24 weeks (which were expected to yield a 25% incidence of PIH) were randomized to receive either 75 mg aspirin daily or a matched placebo (McParland et al 1990). The treated patients were found to have a greatly reduced incidence of early hypertension (0% versus 17%) and proteinuric hypertension (2% versus 19%), whilst reductions in the incidence of PIH (13% versus 25%) and low-birthweight babies (15% versus 25%) did not reach statistical significance. Another group have briefly described a randomized placebo-controlled trial of 150 mg aspirin daily (Trudinger et al 1988). The patients, of unstated parity, were included if an increased umbilical artery systolic/diastolic ratio (fetal) was found at Doppler ultrasound examination between 28–36 weeks, although patients with severe hypertension were excluded. The pregnancy outcomes of 12 patients with extremely abnormal ratios were judged to be unchanged by treatment, whereas those of 34 patients with less markedly abnormal ratios and who received aspirin had an increase in mean birthweight, head circumference and placental weight in comparison with those who received placebo. It is unclear, however, whether there was any difference in fetal growth in each of the randomization groups before treatment was started.

A further description of the use of 75 mg aspirin daily involved treatment of 42 patients with very bad past obstetric histories, including some cases of systemic lupus erythematosus, wherein only 8 of 84 previous pregnancies had resulted in live birth, with growth retardation in each case (Elder et al 1988). Treatment was started in the first trimester in 32 women, and in the second trimester in the other 10. Eighty eight percent of the 38 subsequent aspirin-treated pregnancies resulted in live birth, with growth retardation in 11 (29%). Even allowing for the known trend towards improved pregnancy outcome in subsequent pregnancy with such high-risk patients, these results do suggest a considerable improvement with low-dose aspirin.

Idiopathic intra-uterine growth retardation and pre-eclampsia are thought to share some aspects of pathogenesis (Khong et al 1986), and low-dose aspirin has also been shown in 'small studies' to prevent recurrent IUGR (Wallenburg & Rotmans 1987; Uzan et al 1991) in cases where there has been no hypertension or proteinuria.

Two small prospective studies likewise analysed the effects of aspirin on the incidence of pre-eclampsia. The Birmingham group (Hauth et al 1993) demonstrated a significant decrease in the incidence of pre-eclampsia in the aspirin-treated group (1.7% aspirin-treated versus 5.6% controls; p=0.009). Such a statistically significant effect was not confirmed by the Finnish Study (Odds ratio 0.82; CI 0.33–2.06) (Viinikka et al 1993).

Large, multicentre prospective studies

(i) The **Italian Multicentre Trial (1993)** involved the randomization of 1106 women to either active pharmacological prophylaxis (low-dose aspirin/50 mg daily) or no treatment. The study design did not include the physicians being 'blind' to the treatment used and bias may also have operated in this study as the 'control-group' did not receive a placebo. The outcome of the trial indicated that there was no significant difference in the incidence of pre-eclampsia in the aspirin-treated group (2.12%) compared with the controls (1.88%). However, statification of data based upon parity of subjects was not presented. Similarly, the perinatal deaths in the two groups (2.83% aspirin versus 3.56% control) and the number of babies born with weights below the 10th centile (18.3% aspirin versus 19% control) were not significantly different. It was noted that some patients who were randomized to the no treatment group could have been self-medicating and that this would not have been detected, as no objective test of bias was used (Louden 1993). The number of patients lost to follow-up was significantly greater in the no treatment group (46/523) than those treated with aspirin (18/583; x^2-test, p<0.001).

(ii) The **American study** on the prevention of pre-eclampsia in healthy, nulliparous pregnant women using low-dose aspirin was a multicentre (seven centres), double-blind, placebo-controlled trial (Sibai et al 1993). Overall, 3135 primigravidae were recruited. The active treatment regime involved giving 60 mg of aspirin (1570 subjects) or a placebo (1565 subjects). The benefits, in terms of the prevention of pre-eclampsia in this homogenous group were not demonstrated (4.39% aspirin-treated versus 6.01% controls). However, more worrying was the incidence of perinatal death secondary to abruptio placentæ, which was significantly higher in the aspirin- treated group (0.7% aspirin-treated versus 0.1% placebo; p=0.01). This excess of antepartum haemorrhage may have subsequently been explained by the higher prevalence of cocaine-metabolites in the urine of the aspirin-treated women. Subsequent commentary on this work has indicated that the aspirin-treated group had an abruption rate similar to the 'background' population rate and that the 'placebo' group was significantly lower than this.

(iii) **The Collaborative Low-dose aspirin Study in Pregnancy** was a multicentre study which recruited 9364 pregnant women, between 12–32 weeks gestation from 213 centres in 16 countries between January 1988 and December 1992. This was the largest of the prospective studies to date (de Swiet & Redman 1994) and was a randomized, placebo-controlled trial co-ordinated by the Clinical trial Unit in Oxford. Eligibility for entrance to this study were patents who *in the opinion of the clinician* were at significant risk of pre-eclampsia or IUGR for pharmacological 'anti-platelet' prophylaxis or therapy to be contemplated and with no significant contraindications (i.e. asthma, increased risk of bleeding, allergy to aspirin or likelihood of immediate delivery):

• **Prophylactic entry:** Women with a history of previous pre-eclampsia IUGR, or other risks such as maternal age or family history.
• **Therapeutic entry:** Pregnant women with symptoms and signs of pre-eclampsia or IUGR in the current, index pregnancy.

Seventy-four percent of women were entered for prophylaxis of pre-eclampsia, 12% for prophylaxis of IUGR, and 12% and 3% for treatment of pre-eclampsia and IUGR, respectively. These data indicate one of the weaknesses of the CLASP study–the heterogenous nature of the study group.

Women assigned to treatment were allocated to either 60 mg of aspirin or a matching placebo tablet. This dose was utilized, as it was sufficient to inhibit maternal cyclo-oxygenase-dependent platelet function (Benigni et al 1989) and thought to be of proven efficacy (Wallenburg et al 1986). Data from the study were followed up 6 weeks after the end of this index pregnancy and the following pre-specified outcome measures noted:

1. Development of pre-eclampsia (proteinuric PIH)
2. Duration of pregnancy
3. Crude birthweight and birthweight below 3rd centile for sex and gestation
4. Perinatal loss ascribed to pathology (ie IUGR or pre-eclampsia)
5. Perinatal loss ascribed to therapy.

Overall, the use of low-dose aspirin in pregnant women was associated with a 12% reduction in the incidence of pre-eclampsia as compared with the placebo group: this result did not reach statistical significance (Fig. 2.2). No significant effect was found on the incidence of IUGR or perinatal loss. Low-dose aspirin did, however, reduce the incidence of preterm delivery in this high-risk group (19.7% aspirin versus 22.3% placebo; p=0.015). Interestingly, there was a significant trend (p=0.004) towards

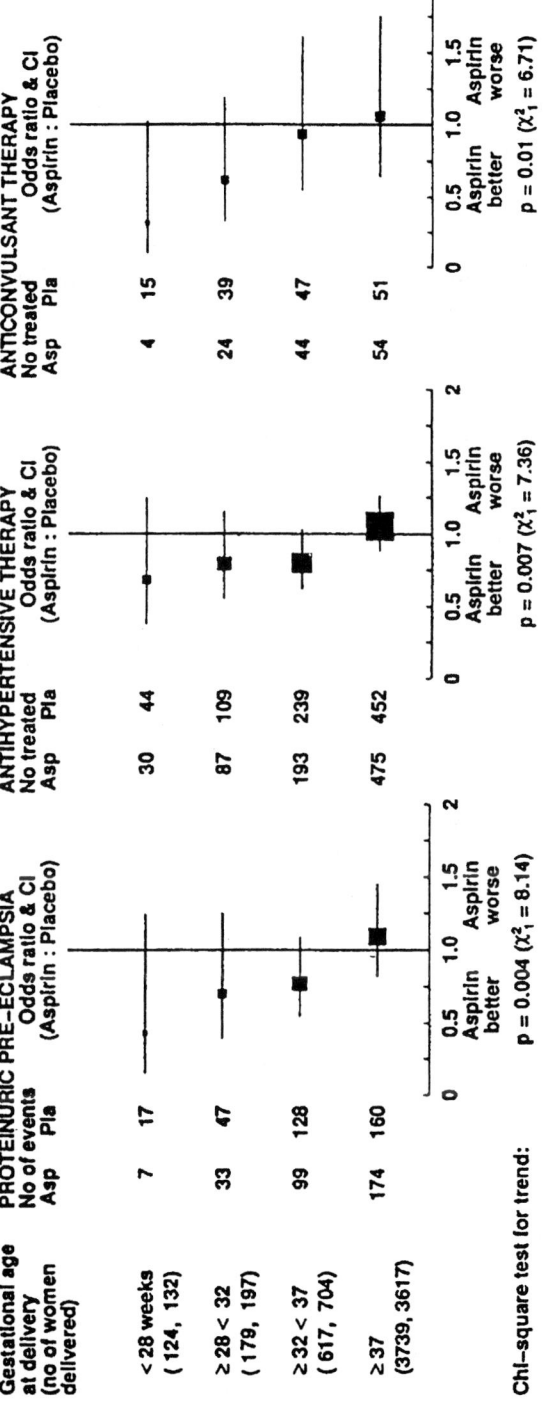

Fig. 2.2   The effect of low-dose aspirin upon the development of pre-eclampsia and the subsequent use of anti-hypertensives and anti-convulsants compared with placebo (CLASP 1994).

progressively higher reductions in pre-eclampsia the more preterm the delivery indicating a possible therapeutic benefit in those who have previously had this disease at an early gestation (Fig. 2.3). There was a similar trend towards decreased use of anti-hypertensive and anti-convulsant therapy in the aspirin-treated group.

The size of the CLASP study made the analysis of data pertaining to complications of therapy interesting and reliable. The aspirin-allocated women had a higher incidence of abruptio placentæ, but this did not reach statistical significance (1.8% aspirin-treated versus 1.5% placebo group). The incidence of unexplained antepartum and postpartum haemorrhages were statistically no different compared to the placebo-treated group, however the percentage of aspirin-treated women who needed postpartum blood transfusion was significantly increased ($p=0.026$; $x^2=4.94$). Of the 9364 pregnant women, 79 had adverse experiences with epidural anaesthesia. Overall, the proportion of these in the aspirin-treated group were no different from the placebo group (3.2% versus 2.4% respectively). In terms

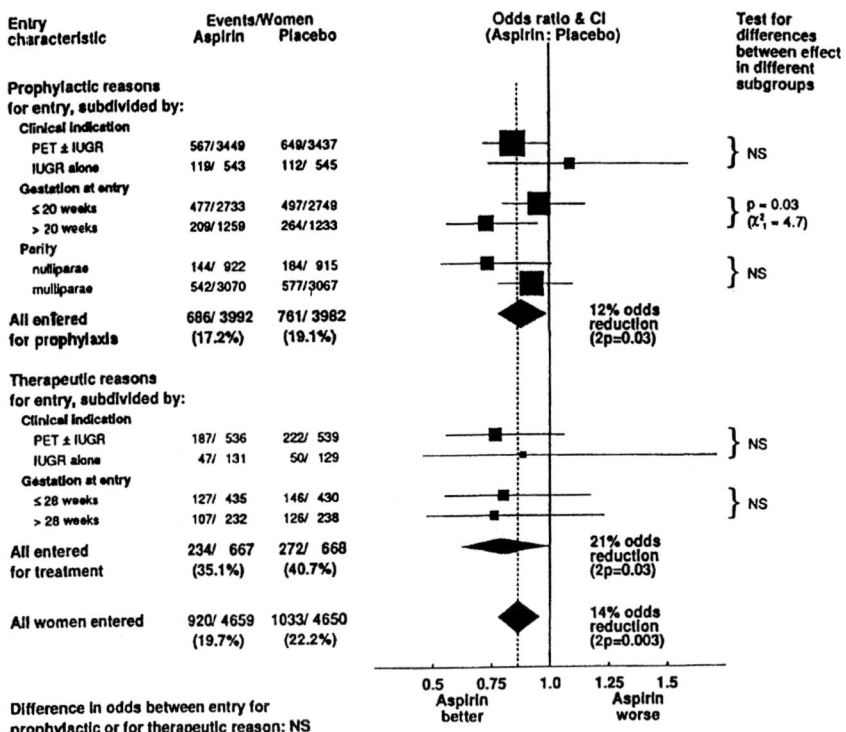

Fig. 2.3 The effect of low-dose aspirin upon the incidence of preterm labour compared with placebo (CLASP 1994).

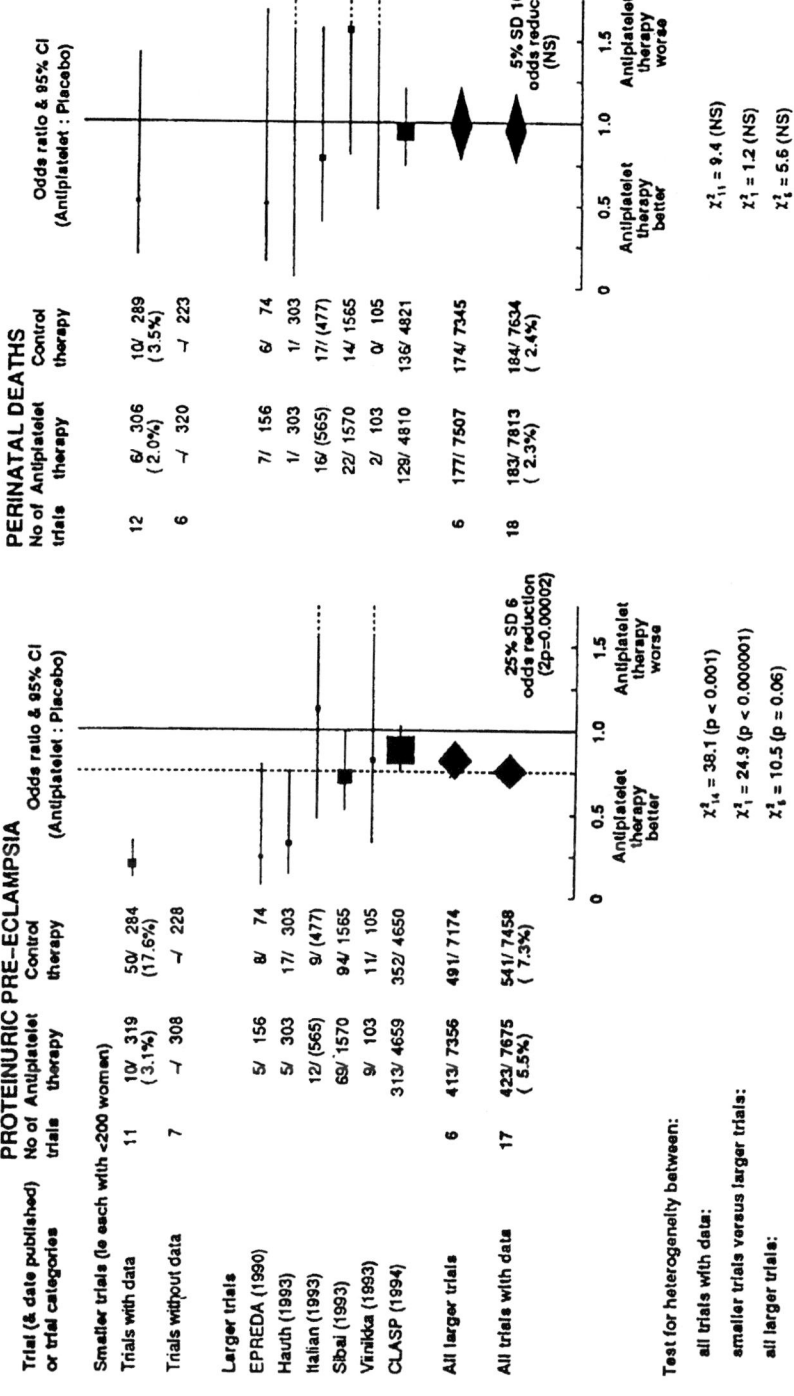

Fig. 2.4   The overview and meta-analysis of all the small and larger prospective double-blind trials using low-dose aspirin. The odds ratios and 95% confidence intervals are presented with respect to the development of pre-eclampsia and perinatal loss (CLASP 1994).

of neonatal haemorrhagic complications, the aspirin-treated group fared no worse than their placebo counterparts. Fewer babies had intraventricular haemorrhages in the aspirin-treated group (although this was not significant) and the total perinatal deaths attributed to haemorrhage were not different in the two groups.

KEY POINTS FOR CLINICAL PRACTICE

1. Low-dose aspirin is a cheap and simple drug that has few recognizable side-effects in either the mother or her baby.

2. The results from small and the larger prospective studies investigating the role of low-dose aspirin in reducing the prevalence of pre-eclampsia are not consistent with each other (test for heterogeneity; p<0.001).

3. The complete 'meta-analysis of all trial 'to-date' indicate that the use of low-dose aspirin in pregnancy would prevent pre-eclampsia in 1 in 100 women treated.

4. The results of available trials do **not** support the widespread and routine prophylactic or therapeutic use of anti-platelet therapy in pregnancy among all women judged to be 'at-risk' of pre-eclampsia or IUGR (Fig. 2.4).

5. The only women in whom the use of low-dose aspirin may be justified are those at especially high risk of early-onset pre-eclampsia (i.e. prior to 32 weeks).

6. It is not possible at present to identify women at especially high risk of early-onset pre-eclampsia prospectively, but those with a previous history might be considered 'at-risk'.

REFERENCES

Ahmed Y, Sullivan M H, Elder M G 1991 Detection of platelet desensitization in pregnancy-induced hypertension is dependent upon the agonist used. Thrombos Haemostas 65: 474–477

Baker P N, Broughton Pipkin F, Symonds E M 1991 Platelet angiotensin II binding sites in normatensive and hypertensive women. Br J Obstet Gynaecol 98 436–440

Baker P N, Kilby M D, Broughton Pipkin F 1992 The effect of angiotensin II on platelet intracellular free calcium concentration in human pregnancy. J Hypertension 10: 55–60

Beaufils M, Uzan S, Donsimoni R, Colau J C 1985 Prevention of pre-eclampsia by early anti-platelet therapy. Lancet 1: 840–842

Benigni A Gregorinin G, Frusca T et al 1989 The effects of low dose aspirin on fetal and maternal generation of thromboxane by platelets in women at risk of pregnancy-induced hypertension. N Eng J Med 321: 357–362

Bergstrom S, Carlson L A Weeks J R 1968 The prostaglandins: family of biologically active lipids. Pharmacol Rev 20: 1–48

Brosens I A, Robertson W B, Dixon H G 1972 The role of spiral arteries in the pathogenesis of pre-eclampsia. In: Wynn R M (ed) Obstetrics & Gynaecology Annual. Appleton-Century-Crofts, New York. pp.

Bucchi F, Bodzenta A, de Gaetano G, Cerlette C 1986 The effects of 1 g of oral or intravenous aspirin upon the urinary excretion of thromboxane B_2 and 6-keto F_{1a} in healthy pregnant subjects. Prostaglandins 32: 691–701

Chesley L C 1978 Hypertensive disorders of Pregnancy. Appleton-Century-Crofts, New York.

CLASP Trial 1994 Collaborative Low dose aspirin study in pregnancy. MRC Collaborative group on Low dose aspirin in pregnancy. Lancet 343: 619–629

Crandon A J, Isherwood D M 1979 Effect of aspirin on incidence of pre-eclampsia. Lancet 1: 1356

Davey D A, MacGillivray I 1986 The classification and definition of the hypertensive disorders of pregnancy. Clin Exp Hyper Hypertens Preg (B). 5: 97–133

DHSS 1994 Report on Confidential Enquires into Maternal Deaths in the United Kingdom; 1988–1990. Her Majesty's Stationery Office, London

Downing I, Sheperd G L, Lewis P L 1982 Kinetics of prostaglandin synthetase in the umbilical artery microsomes from normal and pre-eclamptic pregnancies. Br J Pharmacol 13: 195–198

Elder M G, de Swiet M, Robertson A et al 1988 Low dose aspirin in pregnancy. Lancet 1: 410

EPREDA Trial. Uzam S, Beaufils M, Breast G, Bazin B, Capitant C, Paris J 1991 The prevention of fetal ictordation with low dose aspirin. Lancet 337: 1427–1431

Fitzgerald D J, Entman S S, Mulloy R N, FitzGerald G A 1987 Decreased prostacyclin biosynthesis preceding the clinical manifestation of pregnancy-induced hypertension. Circulation 75: 956–963

Fox S, Burgess-Wilson M E, Heptinstall S, Mitchell J R A 1982 Platelet aggregation in whole blood determined using the Ultra-Flo 100 platelet counter. Thromb Haem 48 327–329

Fox S C, Kilby M D, Sanderson H M, Heptinstall S 1994 Investigations in spontaneous aggregation and platelet responses to streptokinase and adrenaline in Human pregnancy. Platelets 5: 139–144

Gant, N F, Chand S, Worley R J et al 1974 A clinical test useful for predicting the development of acute hypertension in pregnancy. Am J Obstet Gynecol 120: 1–7

Goodlin R C 1983 Correction of pregnancy-related thrombocytopaenia with aspirin without improvement in fetal outcome. Am J Obstet Gynecol 146: 862–864

Goodlin R C, Haslam H O, Fleming J 1978 Aspirin for treatment of recurrent toxaemia. Lancet 2: 51

Greer I A, Walker J J, McLaren M et al 1985 Immunoreactive prostacyclin and thromboxane metabolites in normal pregnancy and the puerperium. Br J Obstet Gynaecol 92: 381–385

Groenendijk R, Trimbos J B M J, Wallenburg H C S 1984 Haemodynamic measurement in pre-eclampsia: preliminary observations. Am J Obstet Gynecol 150: 232–236

Hauth J C, Goldenberg R L, Parker R et al 1993 Low-dose aspirin therapy to prevent pre-eclampsia. Am J Obstet Gynecol 168: 1083–1093

Italian Study of Aspirin in Pregnancy 1993 Low dose aspirin in the prevention and treatment of intrauterine growth retardation and pregnancy-induced hypertension. Lancet 341: 396–399

Khong T Y, De Wolf F, Robertson W B, Brosens I 1986: Inadequate maternal vascular response to placentation in pregnancies complicated by pre-eclampsia and by small-for-gestational-age infants. Br J Obstet Gynaecol 93: 1049–1059

Kilby M D, Broughton Pipkin F, Symonds E M 1992 Calcium, platelets and hypertension. J Hypertension 10: 997–1003

Lewis P J, Boylan P, Friedman I A et al Prostacyclin in pregnancy. Br Med J 282: 1581–1582

Louden K A 1992 Low dose aspirin in pregnancy. Clin Pharm 23: 90–92

Louden K A 1993 Aspirin and pregnancy. Lancet 341: 753

Louden K A, Broughton Pipkin F 1991 Prediction of pregnancy-induced hypertensive disorders by angiotensin II sensitivity and supine pressor test. Br J Obstet Gynaecol 98: 231–233

Louden K A, Broughton Pipkin F, Heptinstall S et al 1990a Maternal low-dose aspirin spares neonatal platelets. Br J Obstet Gynaecol 97: 1162

Louden K A, Broughton Pipkin F, Heptinstall S et al 1990b A longitudinal study of platelet behaviour and thromboxane production in whole blood, in normal pregnancy and the puerperium. Br J Obstet Gynaecol 97: 1108–1114

Louden K A, Broughton Pipkin F, Heptinstall S et al 1991 Platelet reactivity and serum thrombonxane B$_2$ production in whole blood in gestational hypertension and pre-eclampsia. Br J Obstet Gynaecol 98: 1239–1244

Louden K A, Broughton Pipkin F, Symonds E M et al 1992 A randomised placebo-controlled study of the effect of low dose aspirin on platelet reactivity and serum thromboxane B$_2$ production in non-pregnant women, in normal pregnancy and in gestational hypertension. Br J Obstet Gynaecol 99: 371–376

Louden K A, Broughton Pipkin F, Heptinstall S et al 1994 Neonatal platelet reactivity and serum thromboxane B$_2$ production in whole blood: the effect of maternal low dose aspirin. Br J Obstet Gynaecol 101: 203–208

McParland P, Pearce J M, Chamberlain G V 1990 Doppler ultrasound and aspirin in recognition and prevention of pregnancy-induced hypertension. Lancet 1: 1552–1555

Moncada S, Vane J R 1979 Arachidonic acid metabolites and the interaction between platelets and blood vessel walls. N Eng J Med 300: 1142–1147

Moncada S, Grygleewski R, Bunting S, Vane J R 1976 An enzyme isolated from arteries transforms prostaglandin endoperoxides to an unstable substance that inhibits platelet activation. Nature 263: 663–665

Myatt L, Elder M G 1977 Inhibition of platelet aggregation by a placental substance with prostacyclin-like activity. Nature 268: 159–160

Norris L A, Sheppard B L, Bonnar J 1993 Increased whole blood platelet aggregation in normal pregnancy can be prevented in vitro by aspirin and dazmegrel (UK 38485). Br J Obstet Gynaecol 99: 253–257

Norris L A, Sheppard B L, Burke G, Bonnar J 1994 Platelet activation in normotensive and hypertensive pregancies complicated by intrauterine growth retardation. Br J Obstet Gynaecol 101: 209–214

Nuotto E L, Gardin M K, Paasonen M K et al 1984 The effect of acetylsalicyclic acid on plasma thromboxane B$_2$ and platelet aggregation in man. Eur J Clin Pharmacol 25: 313–317

O'Brien J 1968 Effect of salicylates on human platelets. Lancet 1: 779–783

Pederson E B and FitzGerald G A 1984 Dose related kinetics of aspirin: pre-systemic acetylation of platelet cyclo-oxygenase. N Eng J Med 311: 1206–1211

Piper P J, Vane J R 1969 Release of additional factors in anaphylaxis and its antagonism by anti-inflammatory drugs. Nature 223: 29–35

Remuzzi G, Marchesi D, Zoja C et al 1980 Reduced umbilical and placental vascular prostacyclin in severe pre-eclampsia. Prostaglandins 20: 105–110

Roberts J M, Redman C W R 1993 Pre-eclampsia: more than PIH. Lancet 341: 1447–1451

Robertson W B, Brosens I, Dixon H G 1967 The pathological response of the vessels of the placental bed to hypertensive pregnancy. J Pathol Bacteriol 93: 581–592

Roth G J, Majerus P W 1975 The mechanism of the effect of aspirin on human platelets. 1. Acetylation of a particulate fraction protein. J Clin Invest 56: 624–632

Schiff E, Peleg E, Goldenberg M et al 1989 The use of aspirin to prevent pregnancy-induced hypertension and lower the ratio of thromboxane A$_2$ to prostacyclin in relatively high risk pregnancies. N Eng J Med 321: 351–356

Schiff E, Barkai G, Ben-Baruch G, Mashiach S 1990 Low-dose aspirin does not influence the clinical course of women with mild pregnancy-induced hypertension. Obstet Gynecol 76: 742–744

Sibai B, Cartis S N, Thom E et al 1993 Prevention of pre-eclampsia with low dose aspirin in healthy, nulliparous pregnant women. N Eng J Med 329: 1213–1318

Stuart M J, Clark D A, Sunderji S G et al 1981 Decreased prostacyclin production: a characteristic of chronic placental insufficiency. Lancet (i): 1126–1128

Sullivan M F, Elder M 1993 Changes in platelet reactivity following aspirin treatment for pre-eclampsia. Br J Obstet Gynaecol 100: 542–545

de Swiet M and Fryer G 1990 The use of aspirin in pregnancy. J Obstet Gynaecol 10: 467–482

Tateson J G, Moncada S, Vane J R 1977 Effects of prostacyclin on cyclic AMP concentrations in human platelets. Prostaglandins 13: 389–398

Trudinger B, Cook, C M, Thompson R et al 1988 Low-dose aspirin improves fetal weight in umbilical placental insufficiency. Lancet 2: 214–215

Uzan S, Beaufils M, Breart G et al 1991 Prevention of fetal growth retardation with low-dose aspirin: findings of the EPREDA trial. Lancet 337: 1427–1431

Viinikka L, Harkikainen-Sorri A L, Lumme R et al 1993 Low dose aspirin in hypertensive pregnant women; the effect on pregnancy outcome and prostacyclin-thromboxane balance in mothers and the newborn. Br J Obstet Gynaecol 100: 809–815

Wallenburg H C S 1989 Screening for and diagnosis of hypertensive disorders of pregnancy. In: Chalmers I, Enkin M W, Keirse M J N C (eds) Effective care in pregnancy and childbirth. Pub University Press, Oxford, pp 382–402

Wallenburg H C S, Rotmans N 1982 Circulating large platelets and platelet turnover in normotensive and hypertensive pregnancies. Ain Shams University Press, Cairo, pp 283–288

Wallenburg H C S, Rotmans N 1987 Prevention of recurrent idiopathic fetal growth retardation by low-dose aspirin and dipyridamole. Am J Obstet Gynecol 157: 1230–1235

Wallenburg, H C S, Dekker G A, Makovitz J W, Rotmans P 1986 Low-dose aspirin prevents pregnancy-induced hypertension and pre-eclampsia in angiotensin primigravidae. Lancet 1: 1–3

Walsh S W, Behr M J Allen N H 1985 Placental prostacyclin production in normal and 'toxaemic patients'. Am J Obstet Gynecol 151: 110–115

3

The Management of IUGR

R. B. Beattie   M. J. Whittle

True intrauterine growth retardation (IUGR) represents a major risk factor to the fetus and a dilemma for the obstetrician. Appropriate management involves making a diagnosis of IUGR, defining the underlying aetiology, accurately assessing the fetus and placenta and subsequently planning the most appropriate form of surveillance and delivery. In view of the uncertainties a multicentred randomized controlled trial Growth Restriction Intervention Trial (Thornton 1994, personal communication) is currently being conducted in the UK to determine the optimal management of such fetuses.

Despite the vast literature already published on the aetiology, diagnosis and management of IUGR many perinatologists continue to use crude end points, such as birthweight, for gestation, thus confusing the important differences between the statistically small for dates (SFD) baby and the one who has suffered from nutritional deprivation in utero or who, for some other reason, has failed to reach his or her growth potential. In order to make the diagnosis accurate, dating is essential and therefore a detailed menstrual history and, preferably a first or second trimester 'dating' ultrasound examination are crucial. Management consists of making the diagnosis of IUGR, determining the underlying aetiology, excluding fetal abnormality, hypoxia and acidosis, establishing the prospects for safe continued growth in utero, instituting appropriate surveillance and planning delivery. Delay in delivery may lead to the eventual birth of a baby with severe compromise, whilst too early delivery may produce a baby with problems of both prematurity and IUGR. The planning of the optimum timing for delivery based on the perceived fetal condition in such cases is to be addressed by the GRIT protocol (Table 3.1). The eventual development of the IUGR baby may be particularly poor and the long-term implications of the condition as far as later adult health is concerned may be considerable (Barker et al 1990).

DIAGNOSIS OF IUGR

Confounding variables such as maternal height, weight, race, fetal sex and birthweights of previous babies may be corrected for by computer, using

Table 3.1 The scheme devised for the GRIT study indicating the points of uncertainty (?)

Umbilical artery doppler	Gestation Band (completed weeks)				
	24–25	26–27	28–30	31–34	35–36
Reversed EDF	?	?	deliver	deliver	deliver
Absent EDF	wait	?	?	deliver	deliver
EDF severely reduced	wait	wait	?	?	deliver
EDF moderately reduced	wait	wait	wait	wait	?

EDF = end-diastolic velocities

algorithms to derive specific customized growth charts (Wilcox et al 1993), bearing in mind that up to 40% of the variation in birthweight is related to genetic contributions from both the mother and fetus.

Postnatal assessment of even these birthweight centiles should, however, be supplemented by anthropometric studies such as ponderal index ([birthweight (g) × 100]/length^3) (Lockwood & Weiner 1986), midarm circumference: head circumference ratio (MAC: HC) (Georgieff et al 1986; Sasanow et al 1986; Golebiowska et al 1992), and skinfold thickness (Tanner & Whitehouse 1975). These indices are superior in identifying those at maximal risk of neonatal morbidity (Patterson & Pouliot 1987) such as polycythaemia, hypoglycaemia, hypothermia and necrotising enterocolitis and are particularly useful in identifying the IUGR newborn who weighs more than 2500 g.

Those who require more accurate end points for perinatal research should also consider the use of body fat estimation using near infrared interactance (Futrex-5000 1993) and tetrapolar bioelectrical impedance to estimate total body water. The latter technique is relatively simple, inexpensive at under £1000 (Holtain) and closely correlates with the gold standard of body composition analysis (total body water using deuterium) even in preterm neonates.

When patients are referred with suspected IUGR, the ultrasound diagnosis of true IUGR should be based on a number of features apart from a reduced size (e.g. estimated fetal weight <10th centile). Biometric assessment should consist of measurement of the abdominal circumference, head circumference, femur length and cerebellar diameter. The latter is a particularly stable measurement even in profound IUGR (Reece et al 1987). This will give an indication of the relative fetal size and the body proportionality with the classic categorization into symmetrical (type I-20%) IUGR caused by decreased growth potential, and asymmetrical (type II-80%) IUGR associated with restriction of fetal nutrients and oxygen. However, this has limited clinical potential as both patterns overlap in individual cases and the two types probably reflect the timing and duration, rather than the cause of poor growth (Lin & Evans 1984; Lin 1985). A repeat ultrasound examination may be necessary 2 weeks later in order to assess the growth velocity and to avoid the erroneous diagnosis of true IUGR in a fetus which is only constitutionally small but otherwise healthy. Typically a fall of >1.5SD in the AC measurement over this period would be regarded as being indicative of true IUGR (Chang et al 1993). Assessment of liquor volume is equally important with most centres now recognizing the value of the Amniotic Fluid Index measurements as a repeatable and reliable technique.

Key points

1. Accurate gestation
2. Fetal AC <5th centile
3. Fetal growth velocity <1.5SD in 2 weeks
4. Amniotic Fluid Index <5th centile
5. Abnormal umbilical artery Doppler studies.

AETIOLOGY OF IUGR

Having made the diagnosis it is then important to identify the aetiology. This involves taking a detailed obstetric and medical history to identify important risk factors such as advanced maternal age, smoking, alcohol consumption, drug abuse and maternal medical disorders such as hypertension, diabetes and the anticardiolipin syndromes. Enquiry should also be made about possible viral infections (rash and flu-like symptoms) and any history of previous IUGR or structural and chromosomal abnormalities. The maternal blood pressure should be checked and a urinalysis performed. Measurement of the symphysis-fundal height, while useful for screening and monitoring is largely superseded by ultrasound when investigating true IUGR but should be recorded to allow subsequent clinical monitoring of growth (especially to aid the continuation of management in the community) to complement other techniques.

A maternal blood sample should be taken for an infection screen (TORCH and Parvovirus B19), and, if indicated by history and/or findings, an anticardiolipin screen (including lupus anticoagulant). A previously elevated maternal serum alphafetoprotein (MSAFP) in the presence of a structurally normal fetus may indicate a placental origin for the IUGR and is a particularly useful predictor of poor perinatal outcome when levels are elevated in the absence of fetal abnormality. Whilst infection with the TORCH group of viruses is traditionally linked with IUGR there is only strong evidence for rubella (capillary endothelial damage resulting in reduced numbers of normal sized cells), cytomegalovirus (reduced cell number because of cytolysis and localized organ necrosis) (Naeye 1967) and possibly toxoplasmosis (Klein et al 1983; Shi 1992) as causal agents. Overall, about 5% of IUGR is related to infection.

Key points

1. Medical and obstetric history
2. Blood pressure and urinalysis
3. Infection screen (TORCH and Parvovirus)
4. Anticardiolipin and lupus anticoagulant
5. Alphafetoprotein.

ULTRASOUND AND DOPPLER STUDIES IN IUGR

Ultrasound evaluation is appropriate not only to confirm the diagnosis of IUGR, but also to determine the type of IUGR (asymmetrical or symmetrical), exclude fetal and placental abnormalities, and to determine the liquor volume. One may wish to perform Doppler studies to assess the uteroplacental and fetoplacental circulation and the biophysical profile score (BPS) to identify fetal hypoxia. Fetal cardiovascular anomalies such as congenital heart disease, monozygotic twins with a twin–twin transfusion syndrome and a single umbilical artery account for about 1–2% cases of IUGR. The presence of other fetal abnormalities or evidence of congenital infection or hypoxia may prompt invasive diagnostic techniques such as placental biopsy or cordocentesis for karyotyping, virology screening and blood gas analysis.

Multiple pregnancy represents a major risk factory for both IUGR and poor perinatal outcome with up to 20% of twin pregnancies being complicated by IUGR. This may be caused by reduced growth potential with a pattern similar to that seen in singletons with IUGR, poor uterine perfusion, poor maternal nutrition or unique conditions such as the feto–fetal transfusion syndrome. There is some evidence that serial ultrasound biometry, umbilical artery Doppler studies and BPS are complementary in optimizing the outcome in all twin pregnancies (Beattie et al 1993).

Doppler assessment of the umbilical vessels and the uteroplacental vasculature may be important in refining the diagnosis, and certainly reduced diastolic velocities and notching in the uteroplacental artery waveforms correlate well with the development of maternal hypertensive disorders, pre-eclampsia and abnormalities of trophoblast invasion by the spiral arteries. The placental microvasculature responds to a number of pressor agents, such as angiotensin II (Kingdom et al 1993), and it is hypothesized that this leads to eventual obliteration of the vessels. Abnormal umbilical artery Doppler studies indicate high downstream vascular impedance, are associated with IUGR and reduced numbers of tertiary villus vessels (McCowan et al 1989) and are directly related to an increase in the risk and severity of IUGR hypoxia, acidosis and perinatal mortality and morbidity (McParland et al 1991). Comparative studies of serial biometry, umbilical artery Doppler waveform analysis and regional redistribution of fetal blood flow, however, suggest that both isolated and serial biometric assessment remain the most important antenatal diagnostic criteria for true IUGR (Chang et al 1993) but that umbilical artery blood flow studies are superior to antenatal CTGs in pregnancies complicated by IUGR by reducing antenatal admissions for IUGR, fetal distress in labour and caesarean section (Marsal et al 1991).

Key points

1. Biometry (HC, AC, HC:AC, FL, cerebellar diameter)
2. Structural abnormalities
3. Markers for abnormal karyotype
4. Features of infection
5. Biophysical profile score
6. Presentation
7. Multiple pregnancy
8. Doppler (umbilical artery, uteroplacental arteries)
          (?middle cerebral artery, ?renal artery, ?aorta)
9. Liquor (amniotic fluid index).

INVASIVE TECHNIQUES

Karyotype and infection screen

Fetal blood sampling or placental biopsy may be considered for karyotyping though the former procedure is tolerated poorly in true IUGR and sampling on the basis of abnormal biometry alone is probably not justified. Fetal blood should also be sent for infection screen remembering that significant antibody production does not occur until about 22 weeks gestation and thus earlier sampling may produce false negative results. Electron microscopy and polymerase chain reaction (PCR) of amniocentesis samples may be useful in such cases. Lecithin/Sphingomyelin (L/S) ratios and phosphatidyl glycerol may also be measured to evaluate lung maturity and the risks of respiratory distress syndrome (RDS) though this is rarely done nowadays in the UK as the state of the fetal lungs becomes academic if the ultrasound features indicate the need to deliver. Planned delivery before 32 weeks should be preceded by a course of steroids to enhance fetal lung maturity (e.g. IM Dexamethasone 12 mg B.D. for 24 hours).

Key points

1. Blood for karyotype and infection screen (TORCH and Parvovirus)
2. Placental biopsy for karyotype and infection screen.

Assessing fetal hypoxia

Fetal hypoxia may also be indirectly assessed using the BPS or more recently by pulsed Doppler cerebral blood-flow studies. It is thought that increased end diastolic flow velocities in the middle cerebral and carotid arteries correlate with increased cerebral blood flow and shunting away from non-essential fetal vasculature such as the renal and mesenteric arterial systems (Vyas et al 1990). Thus, absolute and sequential changes in the cerebral vessel waveforms and comparison with other vascular beds may prove a useful surrogate measure for fetal adaptation to hypoxia (Di Renzo et al 1992). Supplementary testing includes traditional cardiotocography which may be refined by computerized analysis such as the System 8000, which provides an objective assessment of heart-rate variability (Dawes et al 1992). It is doubtful whether other methods such as contraction stress testing and vibro-acoustic stimulation have much to offer when compared with the BPS and CTG.

Fetal blood gas analysis may also be performed if there is any suspicion of fetal hypoxia (Meizner & Glezerman 1992) though the most appropriate response to an acidotic, hypoxic result is difficult to assess–do you consider delivery to prevent further deterioration or accept that fetal damage is probably already present and intervention will probably lead to a poor fetal outcome? Certainly Nicolini and his colleagues (1990) have suggested that 'since acid-base determination does not predict perinatal outcome in growth-retarded fetuses, fetal blood sampling has a limited role in monitoring fetal wellbeing'.

Key points

1. Blood gases
2. CTG (?computerized analysis)
3. Middle Cerebral Artery Doppler.

TREATMENT OF IUGR

Treatment for IUGR is usually delivery of the fetus by the most appropriate route. Some modalities such as bed rest, oxygen therapy and the administration of nutrients have been criticized, though the treatment of maternal medical disorders such as hypertension and sickle cell disease may be beneficial. The administration of aspirin has received interest of late despite the Cochrane Database of Systematic Reviews of antiplatelet agents for IUGR and pre-eclampsia which failed to show any benefit from therapy. The recent Collaborative Low-dose Aspirin Study in Pregnancy (CLASP 1994) also failed to show any convincing benefits in a heterogenous group of 9364 at-risk women, although the work by McParland and his colleagues (1990), who showed improvement in Doppler blood studies following administration of low-dose aspirin (75 mg daily) to women with abnormal uteroplacental Doppler studies, suggests that careful selection of patients for aspirin therapy may yield some benefits. Patients with the anticardiolipin syndrome will, however, benefit from both aspirin and occasionally steroid or low-dose heparin therapy.

PLANNING DELIVERY

The dilemma surrounding the delivery of the IUGR baby involves the interplay between gestational age and fetal condition. The protocol for the GRIT study emphasizes these difficulties. It needs to be accepted that the very preterm baby in poor condition is most unlikely to be helped by early delivery although even this is uncertain. Planning delivery is based on establishing fetal normality, gestational age, fetal/maternal condition and the aetiology of the IUGR (Table 3.2). Small fetuses with normal growth velocity, liquor volume and Doppler studies should be allowed to progress to term though increased surveillance may be appropriate as features of true IUGR may develop later. Certainly, serial symphysis-fundal height charts and kick charts should be employed as a minimum. Fetuses with true IUGR are at risk and should be delivered if viable and at low risk of RDS. The administration of steroids such as dexamethasone 12 mg BD 24 hours may be advised for fetuses 26–32 weeks gestation or, if available, those with an L/S ratio of <2.0. Obviously if there is evidence of fetal distress, hypoxia or acidosis, immediate delivery may be appropriate. However, the wisdom of intervention in severe IUGR fetuses with evidence of hypoxia and acidosis at gestations of 26 weeks or less should be critically reviewed in the light of their poor prognosis and the additional risk to the mother, should a classical caesarean section be required. When investigations do not fit into a recognizable pattern and, in particular, when liquor volumes are normal or increased in a fetus with poor growth velocity or abnormal Doppler studies, it is particularly important to re-evaluate

Table 3.2 Planning delivery

Size	Normality	Growth/Liquor/Doppler	Gestation	Plan
SGA	Normal	Normal	Any	Allow to term ? increased surveillance
SGA	Normal	Abnormal (TRUE IUGR)	<26 wks	Wait
			26–30 wks	Steroids for 24–48 hours & deliver
			30–32 wks	Steroids 24–48 hours. If L/S ratio available deliver if mature; if not give steroids.
			>32 wks	Deliver
SGA	Normal	INVESTIGATION MISMATCH	Any	Complete investigations before delivery

fetal normality and complete all investigations before contemplating delivery, as these cases are often a result of chromosomal aneuploidy (Rochelson
1989).

INTRAPARTUM AND NEONATAL MANAGEMENT

The second British perinatal Mortality Survey reported a fivefold increase
in the stillbirth rate amongst SFD infants compared with those who were
normally grown, and low Apgar scores and meconium aspiration along
with other manifestations of hypoxia and acidosis in labour are also well
recognized. Close intrapartum surveillance is therefore mandatory, and
indeed serious consideration should be given to caesarean section as the
preferred mode of delivery if antepartum testing suggests severe fetal compromise, especially if the cervix is unfavourable for induction of labour.
For those undergoing labour, continuous electronic fetal heart-rate monitoring is advised with a scalp electrode and early recourse to fetal scalp
sampling for blood-gas analysis and pH.

Regardless of the mode of delivery a senior paediatrician should be present
at delivery to facilitate early and skilled resuscitation and to prevent
meconium aspiration. Suctioning of the oropharnyx by the obstetrician prior
to delivery of the thorax, followed by endotracheal intubation and suctioning
below the cords by the neonatologist is to be recommended if there is any
meconium present (Carson et al 1976).

Early neonatal management should include assessment for fetal abnormality and infection. It is important to monitor and prevent significant
hypothermia and hypoglycaemia especially if the neonate is also premature. When Dextrostix readings are <1.4 mmol/L the neonate should be
treated with early feeding or 10% IV dextrose. Polycythaemia (haematocrit
>65%) can be treated with albumen or partial exchange transfusion if the
haematocrit exceeds 70%. Coagulation defects may also occur and they
should be treated appropriately with fresh-frozen plasma (10 ml/kg) if the
prothrombin time (PT) exceeds 20 seconds or the partial thromboplastin
time (PTT) exceeds 70 seconds.

Long-term follow-up is required for all severely growth retarded fetuses
in view of the well-recognized neurological sequelae and indeed there is
now some suggestion that adult health may also be significantly impaired
in terms of hypertension, cardiovascular disease and carbohydrate intoler-
ance (Barker et al 1990).

Key points

1. Consider caesarean section for severe IUGR
2. Continuous internal electronic fetal monitoring plus fetal scalp
   sampling
3. Senior paediatrician at delivery

4. Prevent meconium aspiration
5. Assess for fetal infection and abnormality
6. Prevent/treat hypothermia, hypoglycaemia, polycythaemia, coagulopathy
7. Long-term follow-up.

REFERENCES

Barker D J P, Bull A R, Osmond C, Simmonds S J 1990 Fetal and placental size and risk of hypertension in adult life. Br Med J 301: 259–262

Beattie R B, McDowell M J, Ritchie J W K 1993 Optimising fetal surveillance in twin pregnancy–The value of biometric, biophysical and Doppler assessment. J Mat Fet Inv 3(1): 53–57

Carson B S, Losey R W, Bowes W A, Simmons M A 1976 Combined obstetric and paediatric approach to prevent meconium aspiration syndrome. Am J Obstet Gynecol 126: 712

Chang T C, Robson S C, Spencer J A, Gallivan S 1993 Identification of fetal growth retardation: comparison of Doppler waveform indices and serial ultrasound measurements of abdominal circumference and fetal weight. Obstet Gynecol 82(2): 230–236

CLASP 1994 CLASP: A randomised trial of low-dose aspirin for the prevention and treatment of pre-eclampsia among 9364 pregnant women. Lancet 343(8898): 619–629

Dawes G S, Lobb M, Moulden M C W, Redman C W, Wheeler T 1992 Antenatal cardiotocogram quality and interpretation using computers. Br J Obstet Gynaecol 99(10): 791–797

Di Renzo G, Luzi G, Cucchia G C et al 1992 The role of Doppler technology in the evaluation of fetal hypoxia. Early Hum Dev 29(1–3): 259–267

Futrex-5000 (1993). Self-Care Products Limited, Amersham, Bucks, England.

Georgieff M K, Sasanow S R, Mammel M C, Pereira G R 1986 Mid-arm circumference/head circumference ratios for identification of symptomatic LGA, AGA and SGA newborn infants. J Pediatr 109: 316–321

Golebiowska M, Ligenza I, Kobierska I et al 1992 Use of midarm circumference: head circumference to estimate gestational age and nutrition staus of newborns. Ginekol Pol 63(5): 221–226

Kingdom J C P, McQueen J, Connell J M C, Whittle M J 1993 Fetal angiotensin II levels and vascular (type I) angiotensin receptors in pregnancies complicated by intrauterine growth retardation. Br J Obstet Gynaecol 100: 476–482

Klein J O, Remington J S, Marcy S M 1983 Current concepts of infections of the fetus and newborn infant. In: Remington J S, Klein J O (eds) Infectious diseases of the fetus and newborn infant, 2nd Edn. W B Saunders, Philadelphia pp 1–26

Lin C C 1985 Intrauterine growth retardation. In: Wynn R M, Norwalk C T, (eds) Obstetrics and Gyanecology Annual 1985. Appleton-Century-Crofts, New York, pp 127–221

Lin C C, Evans M I 1984 Introduction to IUGR In: Lin C C, M I Evans (eds) Intrauterine Growth Retardation: Pathophysiology and Clinical Management. McGraw-Hill, New York, pp 3–15

Lockwood C J, Weiner S 1986 Assessment of fetal growth. Clin Perinat 13(1): 3–35

Marsal K H, Armstrum H H, Axelsson O et al 1991 Umbilical artery velocimetry is more effective than cardiotocography for surveillance of growth retarded fetuses. J Perinat Med 2: 84S

McCowan L, Mullen B, Ritchie J 1989 Umbilical artery blood flow velocity waveforms and the placental vascular bed. Am J Obstet Gynecol 157: 900–902

McParland P, Pearce J, Chamberlain G 1990 Doppler ultrasound and aspirin in the recognition and prevention of pregnancy-induced hypertension. Lancet 335: 1552–1555

McParland P, Steel S A, Pearce J M F 1991 The clinical implications of absent or reversed end-diastolic frequencies in the umbilical artery flow velocity waveforms. Eur J Obstet Gynaecol Reprod Biol 37: 15–23

Meizner I, Glezerman M 1992 Cordocentesis in the evaluation of the growth-retarded fetus. Clin Obstet Gynecol 35(1): 126–137

Naeya R L 1967 Cytomegalovirus disease: The fetal disorder. Am J Clin Pathol 47: 738

Nicolini U, Nicolaidis P, Fisk N M et al 1990 Limited role of fetal blood sampling in prediction of outcome in growth retardation. Lancet 336(8718): 768–772

Patterson R M, Pouliot R N 1987 Neonatal morphometrics and perinatal outcome: Who is growth retarded? Am J Obstet Gynecol 157: 691–693

Reece E A, Goldstein I, Gianluigi G 1987 Fetal cerebellar growth unaffected by intrauterine growth retardation. A new parameter for prenatal diagnosis. Am J Obstet Gynecol 157: 632

Rochelson B 1989 The clinical significance of absent end-diastolic velocity in the umbilical artery waveforms. Clin Obstet Gynecol 43(4): 692–702

Sasanow S R, Georgieff M K, Pereira G R 1986 Midarm circumference and midarm circumference: head circumference ratios: standard curves for anthropometric assessment of neonatal nutrition status. J Pediatr 109: 311–315

Shi D Z 1992 Research on the relation between intrauterine infection and intrauterine growth retardation. Chung Hua Fu Chan Ko Tsa Chih 27(2): 70–72

Tanner J M, Whitehouse R H 1975 Revised standards for triceps and subscapular skinfolds in British children. Archives of Disease in Childhood 50:(2): 142–145

Vyas S, Nicolaides K H, Bower S, Campbell S 1990 Middle cerebral artery flow velocity waveforms in fetal hypoxaemia. Br J Obstet Gynaecol 97: 797

Wilcox M A, Johnson I R, Maynard P V, Smith S J, Chilvers C E D 1993 The individualised birthweight ratio: a more logical approach than birthweight alone. Br J Obstet Gynaecol 100: 342–347

4

Fetal surveillance during labour

P. R. Stone,   H. G. Murray

Labour poses physiological stresses to all fetuses during the transition from the intrauterine to the extrauterine environment. The commonest stress results from the intermittent interruption to maternal–fetal oxygen transfer. Other problems leading to perinatal asphyxia are altered placental gas exchange in abruption or feto-placental growth failure, inadequate maternal perfusion in hypertensive diseases, hypotension, often iatrogenic and impaired maternal oxygenation, for example in severe anaemia or heart disease. Birth asphyxia is defined both clinically and biochemically but there does not appear to be a correlation between the neurological outcome of the fetus and neonatal acidosis unless there are significant, immediate neonatal neurological abnormalities (Nelson & Leviton 1991). Monitoring labour to detect the fetus at risk of developing asphyxia has led to the clinical observations associated with poor fetal outcome, including meconium in the amniotic fluid and bradycardia following contractions, being complemented with forms of electronic and biochemical monitoring aimed at detecting the fetus which is adversely affected by labour.

The methods currently available must be assessed by their ability to address the aims of monitoring the fetus in labour, which are to prevent intrapartum stillbirth, detect umbilical cord problems and signal the development of acidosis caused by the accumulation of lactic acid resulting from anaerobic metabolism. Before discussing the methods of intrapartum fetal surveillance available, it is necessary to define how the fetus may suffer damage from acidosis, and then the fetal response to the stress of labour.

DEFINITION OF PROBLEMS

The various methods and technologies associated with intrapartum fetal surveillance are commonly utilized without a clear understanding of the information they are capable of imparting. The fetus in labour is not a passive onlooker with no threat posed to its existence (Buckell & Wood 1985) and our understanding of the risks to the fetus has only recently been elucidated in terms of biochemical insult and fetal response (Kjellmer 1988). The terms 'fetal distress' and 'fetal asphyxia' have been poorly understood up to now and the use of the terms in both research and clinical practice has led to confusion about what the various forms of surveillance have to offer in terms of predicting imminent fetal damage or death, and therefore what constitutes the need for immediate operative delivery (Steer & Danielian 1994).

The purpose of this chapter is therefore to:

1. Define the threats a fetus may experience in labour
2. Assess the logical objectives of fetal surveillance in labour
3. Discuss the methods of fetal surveillance available in terms of their ability to meet the objectives
4. Discuss a logical approach to the utilization of those methods
5. Briefly look at newer forms of surveillance in the trial phase.

THE THREAT TO THE FETUS IN LABOUR

For some considerable time the understanding of any in-utero threat to a fetus in terms of asphyxia has been clouded by apparently contradictory data. The original concepts of Little (1862) and Haldane (1922) that cerebral palsy and fetal death are caused by hypoxia at the time of delivery have been challenged by epidemiological data showing that by the time labour begins, the majority of cerebral damage has already taken place (Nelson & Ellenberg 1986). More recently, considerable effort has been put into attempts to discredit the use of fetal acid-base status as a means of detection of fetal compromise on the basis of poor correlation between cord artery pH/base excess at delivery and 1 minute Apgar score and/or hypoxic ischaemic encephalopathy. It is surely fanciful to believe that at the moment of delivery all fetal insults have reached a maximum, and that a cord gas will accurately reflect these insults. Despite these contradictions, there is still good evidence that the stresses of labour in terms of metabolic acidosis can lead to cerebral damage and fetal death (Kjellmer 1988), and that such insults are not limited to the pregnancies determined as high risk by virtue of maternal disease or antenatal placental compromise (Sykes et al 1983).

Although the acute events that individually lead to neuronal damage in a fetus are now apparent from animal experiments, a complete understanding of the way these events interact to cause cerebral damage is still incomplete. However, the present state of knowledge can be used to formulate a strategy for intrapartum monitoring.

Fetal neuronal damage, its occurrence and site, are dependent on the degree of the asphyxial insult. The effects of a total cessation of fetal oxygenation, either as a result of total cord occlusion or complete placental abruption, are lesions in the pontine region of the brainstem which almost invariably lead to fetal death. Such insults are obviously rare (Myers et al 1984). Graded (i.e. incomplete) hypoxia or intermittent repetitive cord occlusion leads predominantly to parietal subcortical white matter and basal ganglia necrosis in a distribution similar to that seen in the states of cerebral palsy in the human (Kjellmer 1988). The mechanisms by which the necrosis comes about have been postulated by Kjellmer (1988) and are illustrated in Fig. 4.1. Two groups of compounds are profoundly neurotoxic, namely excitatory amino acids (particularly glutamate) and oxygen radicals released in response to a metabolic acidosis caused by profound hypoxia and are concentrated in the watershed areas of the brain due to the vasoconstriction associated with the lactic acidosis. Glutamate release is triggered by hypoxia, but in a fetus that is able to successfully buffer any production of lactate and maintain cerebral perfusion, the level of glutamate accumulation is insufficient to produce neuronal damage. As the levels of lactate rise in response to the hypoxia and the cerebral vasoconstriction that accompanies a severe metabolic acidosis increases, the accumulating glutamate is able to provide a threat to neuronal integrity, particularly in the low pressure watershed areas of the brain, i.e. the subcortical white matter, the hippocampus and the basal ganglia.

The production of oxygen radicals is more complex. A state of severe metabolic acidosis will cause a disruption of the integrity of cell membranes; the resultant phospholipid release and accumulation providing a substrate store for the production of prostaglandins when the brain is subsequently reperfused as the hypoxic insult resolves. The production of prostaglandins

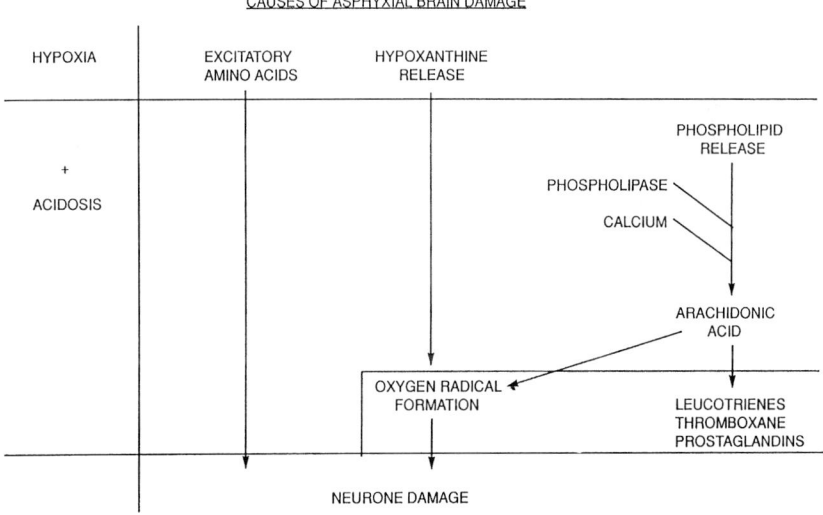

Fig. 4.1 Diagrammatic representation of the theory of causation of asphyxial brain damage as detailed by Kjellmer (1988), (see text for full explanation). Shaded box represents events which follow the reperfusion of the brain with oxygenated blood after a period of hypoxia and metabolic acidosis.

has as an inevitable by-product, oxygen radicals, which are potentially neurotoxic. Oxygen radical production also results from the breakdown of xanthine which accumulates as AMP and is metabolized following a profound hypoxic/acidotic insult. Reperfusion of the areas in which xanthine has accumulated leads to the formation of uric acid, with oxygen radical production again being a by-product.

Recent human observational data would support the animal data conclusions outlined above. Low et al (1988) have shown that worsening levels of buffer base in the umbilical cord of neonates correlates with subsequent neurological deficit as measured in terms of major and minor motor deficits beyond 1 year of age.

Assuming some limitation to the experimental and observational data in terms of numbers, and according to the evidence presented here, the purpose of fetal surveillance in labour must be the detection of lactate accumulation (metabolic acidosis), and the delivery of the fetus at risk of consequent neuronal damage, as well as the detection and delivery of the fetus suffering from an acute and catastrophic asphyxial episode.

FETAL METABOLIC ACIDOSIS – PREVALENCE AND SIGNIFICANCE

Intrapartum stillbirth and cerebral palsy are not common. Asphyxial death in-utero is often accompanied by other contributory factors such as pregnancy-induced hypertension or intrauterine growth retardation, but is probably a factor in between 2 and 5 deaths per 1000 deliveries (Buckell & Wood 1985). Labour complications that result in sublethal neuronal damage in the form that leads to cerebral palsy are rare. The total incidence of cerebral palsy is approximately 2.5 per 1000 deliveries in the western world (Spencer 1989). Of this number, between 8 and 20% may have labour as the cause or part of the aetiology. Most of the neuronal damage associated with cerebral palsy therefore occurs before labour, a finding that explains why most cerebral palsy victims are born with a normal umbilical cord pH.

Cerebral palsy and fetal death are, however, conditions associated with neuronal damage which is complete. There is a third group of fetuses who suffer from hypoxic ischaemic encephalopathy (HIE) that would appear to have had an asphyxial insult but who, after the initial acute episode, survive with little or no impairment. With the inclusion of those with a paediatric diagnosis of mild to moderate HIE, the proportion of children who are at risk of intrapartum HIE amounts to up to 1.0–1.5% of all deliveries in a tertiary unit (Spencer 1989). The total proportion of the population that therefore suffers a degree of asphyxia in a tertiary unit in the developed world is approximately 2%. When a policy for intrapartum monitoring is formulated, this fact, along with the knowledge that 50% of neonatal abnormalities occur in low-risk pregnancies, must be borne in mind.

The final question to be addressed in this section must be: how much lactate can a fetus cope with before the risk of HIE/cerebral palsy/death becomes an issue? Without a doubt, cerebral damage does not occur in all fetuses at the same level of metabolic acidosis. Similarly, there is not a continuum whereby a rising level of lactate will result in a rising level of neuronal damage. Rather, there is a situation whereby the fetus is able to buffer an acid load successfully until the load is so large that cerebral vasoconstriction occurs with all the biochemical sequelae (Kjellmer 1988). The threshold at which this event occurs appears to vary within fetuses of any given gestation, as well as in fetuses with different gestations (Jurgens-van der Zee et al 1979, Huisjes et al 1980).

The concept of a maximum safe lactate load for a given gestation must therefore be developed with the knowledge that for some fetuses the load determined will be an underestimate. Accordingly, Low et al (1988) have looked at a group of term infants and followed them beyond 1 year of age, looking for evidence of cerebral damage associated with lactate load at delivery. Total buffer base levels of less than 34 mmol/L (base deficit 11 mmol/L) appeared to herald the threshold for cerebral dysfunction. It accounted for approximately 2% of the population studied, and fits well with another large study on term infants which has shown that a base deficit of greater than 11 mmol/L is found in 2% of a population delivering at a large tertiary institution (Murray 1992). In units where pH alone is obtained the determination of metabolic acidosis is difficult. Given that the levels of carbon dioxide in the fetus vary widely during labour, and that the fetus is relatively unaffected by carbon dioxide (Khazin et al 1971), determination of pH alone can be misleading in assessing the level of metabolic acidosis and fetal compromise. Data on pH is further confused by the fact that normal fetuses delivered in different units have a different range of umbilical cord pH. This variation possibly reflects differences in second stage policy and maternal position for delivery, and hence neonatal CO_2 levels. The levels of cord artery pH, below which true metabolic acidoses may be found, vary between 7.28 and 7.23 depending on the hospital doing the estimation (Spencer & Ward 1993). These data reinforce the need for all units to utilize the same measure of fetal acidemia to determine fetal compromise. A preference for the detection of buffer base levels is obvious and is based on the evidence presented above. The acid load that the preterm infant (less than 33 weeks) can cope with is as yet uncertain. Without a doubt, the mortality and morbidity of these infants with a buffer base of less than 34 mmol/L would suggest that this level is unsafe. The work of Agustsson & Patel (1988) would suggest that a base deficit of 5 mmol/L (total buffer base of approximately 39 mmol/L) may be the limit of tolerance, at least at the 27–30 week gestation range. Further work is required before absolute rules are applied to these infants, however.

Current fetal surveillance techniques in labour in babies at term should,

therefore, on the basis of the available evidence, be able to detect accumulating lactate and trigger an awareness of a level where the base deficit
approaches 10 mmol/L. At the same time it must be understood that even
with a totally accurate system, only the rate of intrapartum-related problems can be expected to diminish. The rate of cerebral palsy would decrease by a maximum of 20%.

HOW GOOD ARE THE PRESENT-DAY METHODS OF FETAL MONITORING IN THE DETECTION OF FETAL ACIDOSIS?

Current methods of fetal monitoring in labour are largely dependent upon
detecting changes in the fetal heart rate and where this is recorded electronically involve pattern recognition. Although electronic fetal heart rate
monitoring was initially introduced to prevent intrapartum stillbirth, with
increased understanding of the fetal heart rate response to labour, the aim
of monitoring was broadened to detect evidence of fetal stress which may
be associated with cerebral damage.

Clinical methods include intermittent auscultation, detection of the presence of meconium and assessment of the pregnancy for the presence of
factors that may reduce the ability of the fetus to withstand the stress of
labour. The use of risk assessments to predict those fetuses likely to benefit
from intrapartum monitoring has proven to be difficult given that 50% of
neonatal abnormalities thought to be caused by intrapartum events occur
in low-risk pregnancies (Low et al 1981) and evidence that carefully monitored, high-risk pregnancies were less likely to result in the birth of an
asphyxiated fetus than the low-risk group (Sykes et al 1983). Intermittent
auscultation has been used for over a century since it was recognized that
a fetal bradycardia was a pre-terminal event, but even when used by experienced observers with a clear protocol (Boylan 1987) this method is
unable to describe the long-term heart rate variability or the relationship
of fetal heart rate changes to uterine contractions (Hon 1958), features
both now known to be important in predicting whether or not the fetus is
acidaemic.

The often quoted Dublin study comparing electronic fetal heart rate
monitoring with intermittent auscultation (MacDonald et al 1985) was
effectively a trial of these two methods in a low-risk population, given that
babies with meconium, extreme prematurity or absent liquor were excluded
from the trial and in fact only one-third of the intrapartum or neonatal
deaths occurring during the study period were from subjects in this study.
Fewer neonatal seizures occurred in the electronically monitored group,
though there appeared to be little difference between the intermittent auscultation and the electronically monitored groups in labours that were of
less than 5 hours duration. It is interesting to note that the admission test
(Ingemarsson et al 1986) can likewise predict a good outcome if the admission cardiotocograph is normal and delivery occurs within 4 to 5 hours.

The significance of the presence of meconium in labour is similarly controversial and likewise the necessity of rupturing membranes in an attempt to detect the presence of meconium. There would appear to be no evidence to do this where the cardiotocograph is normal. The presence of thick meconium in labour, particularly in association with post-term pregnancy, oligo or anhydramnios and poor fetal growth, has been associated with an increased risk of fetal acidaemia (Boylan 1987), although it has been suggested that meconium as an isolated finding is not correlated with outcome when multiple regression procedures are used, but only with gestation (Steer et al 1989). However, the presence of meconium and fetal heart rate abnormalities are more likely to be associated with acidosis which then increases the risk of meconium aspiration (Boylan 1987).

ELECTRONIC FETAL HEART RATE MONITORING

The initial clinical rationale for this was to reduce the intrapartum stillbirth rate by earlier detection of fetal heart rate abnormalities which precede demises than had been possible with intermittent auscultation, as it had been shown that even in the presence of a cord prolapse there is usually a normal fetal heart rate by 30 seconds after a uterine contraction (Hon 1959). It was shown that fetuses destined to die in labour generally do so with reasonably predictable patterns preceding death, these generally being late or variable decelerations following which there is a baseline tachycardia with reduced long-term variability and finally a terminal bradycardia (Cetrulo & Schifrin 1976). Intrapartum stillbirth is a relatively rare event with an incidence of 1–2 per 1000 labours and it was subsequently suggested that electronic fetal heart rate monitoring could also be used to predict the fetus which was developing acidaemia in labour and enable intervention to occur before damage was sustained owing to the development of acidosis and subsequent asphyxia. However, when used to attempt to achieve this aim, fetal heart rate monitoring has led to an increase in operative intervention in labour without any clear evidence of benefit in terms of neonatal outcomes. This is not surprising given that fetal heart rate changes relate to hypoxaemia, not acidosis.

The relationship between fetal heart rate patterns and the development of acidosis in labour was well described (Beard et al 1971, Tejani et al 1975) before the widespread use of electronic fetal heart rate monitoring in labour and it was shown that even the most abnormal patterns were only likely to be associated with acidosis in around 50% of cases. A brief review of the experimental evidence relating to fetal heart rate decelerations also explains why fetal heart rate monitoring, used uncritically without an understanding of the mechanisms of heart rate changes, is likely to lead to misinterpretation of the information being provided by the cardiotocograph. As a generalization, fetal heart rate changes are caused by an increase in fetal parasympathetic activity. Slowing of the fetal heart may be a result of a number of factors, including increase in cerebro spinal fluid pressure which may be caused by head compression leading to early decelerations. An increase in the umbilical venous pressure from cord compression may also lead to early decelerations, as well as variable decelerations, depending on the degree of compression and whether the artery or the vein are both compressed. When both vessels are compressed there is an increase in vagal stimulation from baroreceptors owing to an increase in the blood pressure (Itskovitz et al 1983). Hypoxemia will lead to stimulation of chemoreceptors with a complex response: parasympathetic stimulation leading to an increase in vagal tone; sympathetic stimulation will cause peripheral vasoconstriction but umbilical perfusion will be maintained. Later, with increasing hypoxemia, there will be fetal catecholamine release (Gu et al 1985) which may overcome the vagally induced bradycardia leading to a rebound tachycardia. Hence, accelerations and a rising baseline are indicative of a fetal stress response in labour and need to be viewed with caution.

Deceleration during contractions, therefore, indicate transient hypoxemia but there is no evidence that hypoxemia alone is harmful to the fetus. However, a time-related association between hypoxemia and the development of acidemia has been shown (Fleischer et al 1982) and a base deficit will develop if lactate accumulates. It is important to note that the early descriptions of outcomes after monitoring were in association with acidemia (Kreb et al 1979) and although the fetal heart rate was a sensitive indicator of hypoxemia it could not be used alone to detect acidemia. Basic physiology shows that hypoxaemia leads to the production of metabolic acids, in particular lactate and pyruvate, and a metabolic acidosis is the best indicator of oxygen debt. Initially the production of metabolic acids is buffered and it is the consumption of buffers to restore the pH towards normality that leads to the development of a base deficit.

It would appear that only 2% of labours are associated with the development of a significant base deficit leading to asphyxia (Low 1993) defined as an umbilical arterial base deficit of 11 mmol/L. Yet only about 40% of cardiotocographs in the first stage of labour are not complicated by decelerations or other abnormalities.

In addition to understanding the reasons for fetal heart rate changes it is also important to be clear and consistent about the definitions of fetal heart rate patterns if these are to be used to predict the likelihood of fetal acidemia and the need to determine the acid-base status of a particular fetus in labour. A reasonable consensus now exists on the definition of the heart rate patterns and these are listed in the accompanying table (Table 4.1) and the categorization of these patterns into normality or otherwise has been agreed (FIGO 1987). A number of points need to be noted when these classifications are used. The interpretation of the fetal heart rate pattern needs to be consistent, include the clinical context, the stage of labour and the contraction or tocographic pattern once it has been determined that the recording of the heart rate is technically adequate. The definitions used for

Table 4.1   Defining the intrapartum CTG

Baseline fetal heart rate	110–160 beats per minute
Long-term variability	5–25 beats per minute (taken over 1 minute over the most reactive part of the record with a stable baseline)
Tachycardia	A sustained rise in heart rate > 160 beats per minute
Bradycardia	A sustained fall in heart rate < 100 beats per minute for > 3 minutes
Unreactive ('flat') trace	Loss of normal long-term variability > 35 minutes
Acceleration	Rise in heart rate ≥ 15 beats per minute for ≥ 15 seconds
Deceleration	Fall in heart rate ≥ 15 beats per minute for ≥ 15 seconds
Early deceleration	Deceleration where the lowest point of the heart rate occurs within 20 seconds of the peak of the contraction
Late decelerations	Decelerations where the lowest part of the heart rate occurs more than 20 seconds after the peak of the contraction. There must be ≥ 3 or more such decelerations following consecutive contractions for a diagnosis of late decelerations to be made.
Variable decelerations	All decelerations not fitting the definitions of early or late

Comments on definitions.
The baseline rate in labour is higher than that quoted by FIGO (1987) as the baseline rate is higher than that observed antenatally because of the normal stress response of labour. There is little evidence that rates up to 160 beats per minute are associated with an adverse outcome, whereas baseline rates greater than 160 and certainly 170 beats per minute are clearly abnormal.
The long-term variability is the only accurate term to describe the fluctuations of the heart rate produced on the monitor. The normal amplitude is 5–25 beats per minute, though in episodes of quiet fetal activity rates less than 5 beats per minute for less than 40 minutes are normal and not associated with adverse outcomes. Modern equipment with auto-correlation does not enable assessment of beat-to-beat variation. This terminology is of no value and increasing the paper speed to more than 1 cm per minute has not been shown to enhance the information obtained from the variability in the baseline heart rate. Baseline variability has also been termed band width. Increased baseline variability of more than 25 beats per minute has been termed saltatory variability. There would appear to be consensus that to qualify for the term deceleration the duration of fetal heart rate slowing needs to be 15 seconds; the original 10 seconds would appear to be too short. This then becomes consistent with a 15 second duration of a rise in the heart rate being termed an acceleration. It is noted that none of the definitions now include a depth of deceleration as this bears no relationship with outcome.

the intrapartum fetal heart rate patterns differ from those used antenatally because of a number of factors. First, in labour the fetus is stressed to varying degrees and is likely to exhibit catecholamine release which will influence the heart rate. Second, fetal behaviour influences the fetal heart rate pattern in labour. The rest-activity cycles are frequently present but are of a shorter duration in most cases than that seen antenatally (Spencer & Johnson 1986) and in quiet episodes the fetal heart rate variability may well be reduced to less than 5 beats per minute. Third, decelerations caused by fetal hypoxia, secondary to interruption of the maternal-fetal oxygen exchange during contractions, are not a normal finding in the antenatal CTG.

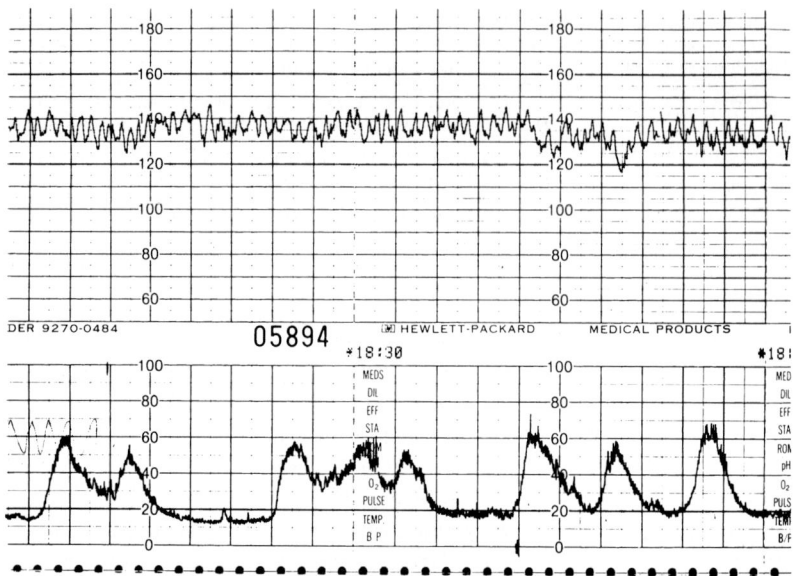

Fig. 4.2   Sinusoidal type 1 pattern (normal outcome).

AIDS IN INTERPRETING THE CTG

Some points are worth noting in interpreting changes in the CTG. Early decelerations are due to fetal head or cord compression as discussed earlier. Should the fetal heart rate fall below 100 beats per minute placental perfusion becomes ineffective and this explains why early decelerations may result in fetal acidaemia. The presence of a rising baseline heart rate, loss of long-term variability or loss of shouldering can all be signs of increasing acidosis and require an assessment of fetal acid-base status, especially if early decelerations are repetitive and have been present for over 45 minutes. Late decelerations are said to occur when there have been 3 or more such decelerations following consecutive contractions. Late decelerations indicate fetal hypoxia where the PO_2 has fallen to less than 1.5 kPa. It must be noted that the depth of these decelerations is often within the normal baseline heart rate range and bears no relationship to the level of fetal hypoxia or development of acidosis. Variable decelerations are best thought of as all decelerations not fitting the definitions of early or late, and may or may not be associated with hypoxia.

Another pattern which has been described is the sinusoidal one of which there would appear to be two types. Sinusoidal type 1 is a saw tooth pattern (Fig. 4.2) which may be a consequence of a small fall in the fetal PO_2. It is thought to be related to a reduction in fetal sympathetic tone, but unless other changes supervene it is generally benign. Associations with fetal haemorrhage have been described, but in general there is no good evidence that this is highly predictive of feto-maternal haemorrhage. The sinusoidal type 2 pattern (Fig. 4.3) is the pattern as described by FIGO (1987). The baseline varies like a smooth sine wave with a frequency of less than 6 cycles per minute and an amplitude of at least 10 beats per minute. This is a very abnormal pattern associated with acidosis and asphyxia and is generally pre-terminal. Clearly then, from an understanding of the production of heart rate changes in labour, assessment of fetal acid-base status based on the fetal heart rate will be imprecise. It is not entirely clear whether classification of CTGs into normal, suspicious and ominous, or pathological (FIGO 1987) enhances the clinical decisions rather than describing the specific CTG abnormalities and relating these to the likelihood of fetal acidosis. However, a detailed study comparing normal, including early decelerations, with all other abnormalities did show that categorizing the CTG patterns in this way was helpful (Steer et al 1989). Abnormalities in the baseline rate or long-term variability without decelerations in the Dublin study were associated with a 21% incidence of acidosis, whereas where decelerations were present there was a 27% incidence of acidosis. There is evidence that certain fetal heart rate patterns (Shields & Schifrin 1988) and acidemia (Low et al 1988) lead to adverse outcomes, but the relationship between fetal heart rate changes and the likelihood of acidemia needs to be examined. There is now reasonable agreement on the range of pH, blood gas and acid-base values in labour and at delivery. The range of values (derived from multiple sources) would

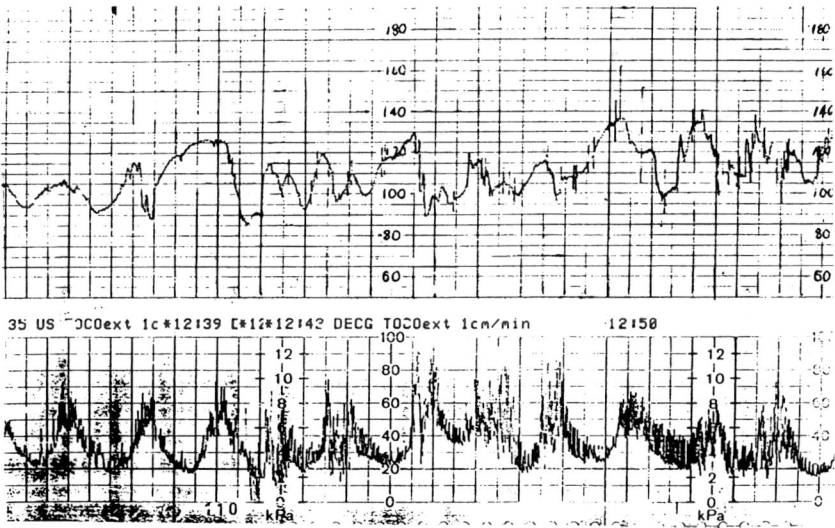

Fig. 4.3 Synusoidal type 2 pattern (intrapartum abruption).

generally be accepted to be pH 7.20–7.34 and base deficit down to 8 mEq/ L in labour. Normal umbilical arterial values have a range of pH 7.23– 7.29 with a base excess down to 8 mEq/L. A number of authors have studied the relationship between fetal heart rate patterns and likelihood of acidosis (Beard et al 1971; Tejani et al 1975). What is clear is that a normal fetal heart rate with normal baseline and long-term variability and no decelerations, even in a high risk group (Tejani et al 1975), is associated with less than a 10% chance of a pH in labour of less than 7.25. Where the CTG is abnormal the chance of acidosis is increased (Steer et al 1989), but even with the pattern most likely to be associated with acidosis, i.e. a complicated baseline tachycardia (Beard et al 1971), the sensitivity is only 50%. It is not possible in the individual case to determine the likelihood of acidosis from the CTG alone.

Other factors may enhance the prediction of acidosis in the presence of CTG abnormalities. The controversy surrounding the significance of meconium has already been discussed. There would appear to be a threefold increase in the relative risk of an Apgar score of less than 7 at 1 and 5 minutes and acidosis when there are meconium and CTG abnormalities (Steer et al 1989).

In the presence of decreased long-term variability, fetal stimulation resulting in a return to a normal pattern is generally associated with a non-acidemic fetus (Clark & Paul 1985) which has led to the suggestion that fetal heart rate assessment may be superior to scalp pH in detecting the non-compromised fetus. Use of vibro-acoustic stimulation to stimulate the fetus (Ingemasson et al 1988) has not been subjected to a randomized trial and may be harmful to the fetus (Mulder et al 1987). In general, fetal heart-rate monitoring has high sensitivity but poor specificity for acidosis and only by assessment of fetal acid-base status will unnecessary operative intervention be avoided. Combining fetal heart-rate monitoring with fetal blood sampling can avoid any increase in the Caesarean section rate (MacDonald et al 1985).

SECOND STAGE OF LABOUR

Interpretation of the fetal heart rate in the second stage of labour is difficult given the high incidence of variable decelerations in well over a third of cases, or even an unclassifiable pattern in 36% (MacDonald et al 1985). In the expulsive phase of the second stage the fetus becomes progressively acidotic with increasing duration of the second stage (Wood et al 1973) and a number of fetal heart-rate abnormalities have been associated with acidaemia (Gilstrap et al 1984; Katz 1987) or increasing umbilical arterial lactate (Piquard et al 1988). Particular patterns which are consistently very abnormal are a decreased baseline heart rate of less than 90, often with decreased long-term variability, decreased baseline rate less than 90 with marked accelerations during contractions (Piquard et al 1988) and loss of variability and/or a fetal tachycardia. In the presence of a fetal heart-rate abnormality in the second stage, unless delivery is imminent, assessment of pH is more appropriate than encouraging expulsive efforts which may further compromise the fetus.

MEASUREMENT OF FETAL ACID-BASE STATUS

The preceding discussion has shown that an abnormal fetal heart rate pattern only serves as an indicator of acidaemia. However, acidaemia usually develops after the CTG becomes abnormal. This is more predictive of acidaemia than abnormalities of the T/QRS ratio of a fetal ECG (MacLachlan et al 1992). Determination of fetal acid-base status is necessary to confirm whether or not the abnormal heart-rate pattern is associated with acidemia. The pH and base deficit are the most useful values to assess fetal condition (Blechner 1993). The PO_2 values may not change with large reductions in fetal oxygen reserves and are not reliable in assessing the fetal condition, but do give an indication of the quality of the blood sample or its analysis. The PCO_2 indicates whether there is a respiratory component to any acidosis present, as a low pH may be a consequence of respiratory or metabolic acidosis.

The base deficit, determined from a nomogram using pH and PCO_2 or bicarbonate concentration, indicates that the production of metabolic acids has depleted the fetal buffering capacity. Changes in the base deficit are prolonged because of poor placental permeability to bicarbonate.

The diagnosis of fetal asphyxia requires blood gas and acid-base measurements demonstrating significant metabolic acidosis, i.e. a buffer base < 34 mmol/L or a base deficit > –11 mEq/L (Low 1988, Johnson et al 1990). Not all fetuses adversely affected by labour have suffered from impaired gas exchange leading to hypoxia, acidosis, acidemia and asphyxia. Infection, drugs administered to mother, haemorrhage or trauma may all necessitate resuscitation at delivery. Assessment of acid-base balance has a limited role in these situations (Lissauer & Steer 1986). Conversely, even when acid-base balance is abnormal, gestation, birth weight and exposure to meconium or trauma will determine the significance and importance of this (Steer 1987).

FETAL BLOOD SAMPLING IN LABOUR

Contrasted with the CTG which is easy to perform but difficult to interpret, fetal blood sampling whilst relatively easy to interpret is more challenging to perform; this being a major disincentive to its use. Fetal blood sampling is best performed with the woman in a left (or right) lateral position. It is important to exclude amniotic fluid (which is alkaline) and meconium from the sample by applying sufficient pressure to the scalp with the amnioscope. Modern analysis equipment requires only a 30–

40 μL/sample. Failure of the fetal scalp to bleed despite good sampling technique is abnormal and suggests that the fetus is peripherally vaso-constricted. A reactive response on the CTG to scalp stimulation is highly predictive of a non-acidotic fetus (Clark & Paul 1985).

In the presence of continuing or evolving CTG abnormalities one fetal blood sample will not suffice. Acidosis occurring in response to hypoxia can take more than 90 minutes to develop in a normally grown fetus (Fleischer 1982), but a poorly grown fetus will become acidotic more quickly (Lin 1980). As obtaining and analysing a fetal blood sample generally re-quires 30 minutes, the need for frequent sampling in abnormal labours must be balanced by the ability to achieve this in practice.

There are situations where attempting fetal blood sampling is neither necessary nor wise. Fetal heart rate changes secondary to iatrogenic fac-tors such as maternal hypotension, or over administration of oxytocin are best corrected by treating the cause. A fall in fetal pH is a late event in chorioamnionitis and many fetuses will have a normal pH despite CTG abnormalities (Hauth et al 1985). Similarly, clear CTG abnormalities in early labour, particularly with the presence of meconium and when the stage of cervical dilatation is such that blood sampling is not practical, warrant delivery rather than incurring delays attempting a blood sample.

FUTURE TRENDS IN INTRAPARTUM MONITORING

The intrinsic problems with the present-day methods of intrapartum monitoring, namely the fact that the CTG is a screening, but not a diagnostic, tool and a fetal blood sample is an intermittent, but not a con-tinuous measure, has led to the search for more accurate methods of moni-toring. The approach to these new methods has been twofold. Given the natural conservatism of obstetric caregivers and the proven screening ca-pabilities of the CTG, most new techniques utilize the CTG as their basis and add further analysis of fetal signals to improve its diagnostic capabili-ties in the realm of fetal stress, fetal distress, and impending fetal asphyxia. Other technologies attempt to stand alone in that they do not utilize any CTG analysis and are being assessed as new versus old technology with a sometimes arbitrary end point in the neonate to denote superiority of one over the other. It is the end-point determination, commonly based around the discredited Apgar score and cord pH level, that has hampered a true analysis of any given technology. As suggested here, perhaps an outcome related to the determination of the rates of HIE, asphyxia due to severe intrapartum metabolic acidosis and an analysis of the LUSCS rate may be of benefit. Trials with such end points are rare.

FETAL ELECTROCARDIOGRAM (FECG)

Two groups are looking at the FECG waveform. Westgate et al (1992) has produced a study of the CTG versus CTG + T-wave estimation and have shown that the T-wave can diminish the need for blood sampling in fetuses with normal or intermediate tracings, i.e. aid the inexperienced CTG assessor. The abnormal CTG, however, often appeared to have a raised T-wave which required a blood sample to determine fetal condition. This finding is not surprising when the strong relation between T-wave height and adrenaline levels in the fetus is taken into account (Murray 1992), increased adrenaline being a sign of fetal stress but not necessarily distress. Recent data suggests that the change in T-wave height rather than absolute T-wave height correlates with fetal condition (Westgate 1993, personal communication). This finding which is in agreement with others (Murray 1992; Khazin et al 1971), throws some doubt on the T-wave studies. A recent report of discrepancy in the determination of the T-wave height owing to signal isolation and analysis (Spencer & Ward 1993) suggests that further work is necessary before the place of the T-wave in clinical monitoring is finalized.

The second group investigating the FECG waveform have analysed all sections of the signal to ascertain its use in the determination of fetal condition (Murray 1992). With the aim of using the easier-to-isolate time intervals like P-R interval, that group are in the final stages of completing animal and observational studies to determine any possible role in intrapartum monitoring.

Pulsed oxymetry and near infrared spectroscopy (NIRS) are also the subjects of work into intrapartum monitoring and at present are being used in conjunction with the CTG. Often heralded as forms of noninvasive fetal monitoring, the term 'noninvasive' is purely relative given that probes are required to contact the fetal skin, preferably in a region without hair, by being passed into the vagina and through the cervix to get a signal. The theoretical advantage of the analysis is that the scalp oxygen saturation (SaO_2) measured by oxymetry and the oxy- to deoxy-haemoglobin ratios of the fetal cerebral circulation measured by NIRS should reflect not only oxygen levels but also levels of acidemia. The relative roles of lactate and carbon dioxide in the final estimation of oxygen availability, and the relationship between monitoring and the final outcomes in labour are not yet completely determined.

KEY POINTS FOR CLINICAL PRACTICE

1. Fetal surveillance in labour requires an understanding of what the methods can achieve.

2. All fetal surveillance methods are tests which must be interpreted in the clinical context.

3. Interpretation of the cardiotocograph requires careful inspection using accepted definitions.

4. Fetal heart rate changes (other than normal patterns) reflect hypoxemia, not acidosis. Define the pattern, then decide on the likelihood of acidosis.

5. Asphyxia is due to acidaemia.

6. Fetal pH and acid-base deficit are required to confirm acidaemia and a metabolic acidosis owing to the consumption of buffers, and prevent unnecessary Caesarean sections for CTG abnormalities.

7. Umbilical cord blood gas and acid-base assessment will prevent subsequent neonatal events being attributed to birth asphyxia when this was not the case.

8. A reactive admission test is highly predictive of a normal outcome, especially if delivery occurs within 5 hours.

9. In certain circumstances fetal scalp sampling is inappropriate and delivery should be expedited. Usually these situations are obvious clinically.

REFERENCES

Agustsson P, Patel N 1988 Intrapartum asphyxia and subsequent disability. Ballières Clin Obstet Gynaecol 2: 167–186

Beard R W, Filshie G M, Knight C A et al 1971 The significance of the changes in the continuous fetal heart rate in the first stage of labour. J Obstet Gynaecol Br Cmmwlth 78: 865–881

Blechner J N 1993 Maternal-fetal acid-base physiology. Clin Obstet Gynecol 36: 3–12

Boylan P 1987 Intrapartum fetal monitoring. Baillière's Clin Obstet Gynaecol 1: 73–95

Buckell E W C, Wood B S B 1985 Wessex perinatal mortality survey. Br J Obstet Gynaecol 92: 550–558

Cetrulo L, Schifrin B S 1976 Fetal heart rate patterns, preceding death in utero. Obstet Gynecol 48: 521–527

Clark S L, Paul R H 1985 Intrapartum fetal surveillance: The role of fetal scalp blood sampling. Am J Obstet Gynecol 153: 717–720

FIGO News 1987 Guidelines for the use of fetal monitoring. Int J Gynaecol Obstet 25: 159–167

Fleischer A, Schulman H, Jagani N et al 1982 The development of fetal acidosis in the presence of an abnormal fetal heart rate tracing. 1. The average for gestational age fetus. Am J Obstet Gynecol 144: 55–60

Gilstrap L C, Hauth J C, Toussaint S 1984 Second stage fetal heart rate abnormalities and neonatal acidosis. Obstet Gynecol 63: 209–213

Gu W, Jones C T, Parer J T 1985 Metabolic and cardiovascular effects on fetal sheep of sustained reduction of uterine blood flow. J Physiol 368: 109–129

Haldane J S 1922 In Respiration. Yale University Press, New Haven, pp 23–24

Hauth J C, Gilstrap L C, Hankins G D V et al 1985 Term maternal and neonatal complications of acute chorioamnionitis. Obstet Gynecol 66: 59–62

Hon E H 1958 The Electronic Evaluation of the Fetal Heart Rate. Preliminary Report. Am J Obstet Gynecol 75: 1215–1230

Hon E 1959 The fetal heart rate patterns preceding death in utero. Am J Obstet Gynecol 78: 47–56

Huisjes H J, Touwen B C L, Hoekstra J et al 1980 Obstetrical-neonatal neurological relationship. A replication study. Eur J Obstet Gynecol Reprod Biol 10: 247–256

Ingemarsson I, Arulkumaran S, Ingemarsson E et al 1986 Admission test: a screening test for fetal distress in labour. Obstet Gynecol 68: 800–806

Ingemarsson I, Arulkumaran, Paul R M et al 1988 Fetal acoustic stimulation in early labour in patients screened with the admission test. Am J Obstet Gynecol 158: 70–74

Itskovitz J, La Gamma E F, Rudolph A M 1983 The effect of reducing umbilical blood flow on fetal oxygenation. Am J Obstet Gynecol 145: 813–818

Johnson J W C, Richards D S, Wagaman R A 1990 The case for routine umbilical cord acid-base studies at delivery. Am J Obstet Gynecol 162: 621–625

Jurgens-van der Zee A D, Bierman-van Eendenburg M E C, Fidler V J et al 1979 Preterm birth, growth retardation and acidaemia in relation to neurological abnormality of the newborn. Early Hum Dev 3: 141–154

Katz M, Lunenfeld E, Meizner I et al 1987 The effect of the duration of the second stage of labour on the acid base state of the fetus. Br J Obstet Gynaecol 94: 425–430

Khazin A F et al 1971 Biochemical studies of the fetus v fetal pCO_2 and apgar scores. Obstet Gynecol 38: 535–545

Kjellmer I 1988 Prenatal and intrapartum asphyxia. In: Levene M, Bennet M, Punt J (eds) Fetal and Neonatal Neurology and Neurosurgery. Churchill Livingstone, London, pp 357–369

Krebs H B, Petres R E, Dunn L J et al 1979 Intrapartum fetal heart rate monitoring. 1. Classification of prognosis of fetal heart rate patterns. Am J Obstet Gynecol 133: 762–780

Lin C C, Moawad A H, Rosenow P J et al 1980 Acid-base characteristics of fetuses with intrauterine growth retardation during labour and delivery. Am J Obstet Gynecol 137: 553–559

Lissauer P J, Steer P J 1986 The relation between the need for intubation at birth, abnormal cardiotocograms in labour and cord arterial blood gas and pH values. Br J Obstet Gynaecol 93: 1060–1066

Little W J 1862 On the influence of abnormal parturition, difficult labour, premature birth, and asphyxia neonatorum on the mental and physical conditions of the child, especially in relation to defomities. Trans Obstet Soc, London, 3: 293

Low J A 1988 The role of blood gas and acid-base assessment in the diagnosis of intrapartum fetal asphyxia. Am J Obstet Gynecol 159: 1235–1240

Low J A 1993 The relationship of asphyxia in the mature fetus to long term neurological function. Clin Obstet Gynecol 36: 82–90

Low J A, Karchmar J, Broekhoven L et al 1981 The probability of fetal metabolic acidosis during labor in a population at risk as determined by clinical factors. Am J Obstet Gynecol 141: 941–951

Low J A, Galbraith R S, Muir D W et al 1988 Motor and cognitive deficits after intrapartum asphyxia in the mature fetus. Am J Obstet Gynecol 158: 356–361

MacDonald D, Grant A, Sheridan-Pereira M et al 1985 The Dublin randomised controlled trial of intrapartum fetal heart rate monitoring. Am J Obstet Gynecol 152: 524–539

MacLachlan N A, Spencer J A D, Harding K et al 1992 Fetal acidaemia, the cardiotocograph and the T/QRS ratio of the fetal ECG in labour. Br J Obstet Gynaecol 99: 26–31

Mulder H H, Visser G H A, Wit H P et al 1987 Effects of vibroacoustic stimulation on fetal behaviour. Abstract C17, 14th Annual Meeting, Soc Study Fetal Physiol, Groningen

Murray H G 1992 Evaluation of the fetal electrocardiogram. MD Thesis, University of Nottingham, Nottingham, UK

Myers R E, de Courten-Myers G M, Wagner K R 1984 Effect of hypoxia on fetal brain. In: Beard R W, Nathanielsz P W (eds) Fetal Physiology and Medicine, 2nd ed. Butterworths, London, 419–458

Nelson K B, Ellenberg J H 1986 Antecedents of cerebral palsy. N Engl J Med 315: 81–96

Nelson K B, Leviton A 1991 How much of neonatal encephalopathy is due to birth asphyxia? Am J Dis Child 145: 1325–1331

Piquard F, Hsiung R, Mettauer M et al 1988 The validity of fetal heart rate monitoring during the second stage of labor. Obstet Gynecol 72: 746–751

Shields J R, Schifrin B S 1988 Perinatal antecedents of cerebral palsy. Obstet Gynecol 71: 899–905

Spencer J A D 1989 Intrapartum hypoxia, birth asphyxia and handicap. In: Spencer J A D (ed) Fetal Monitoring. Castle House Publications, Kent, pp 228–232

Spencer J A D, Johnson P 1986 Fetal heart rate variability changes and fetal behavioural cycles during labour. Br J Obstet Gynaecol 93: 314–321

Spencer J A D, Ward R H T 1993 Intrapartum monitoring. RCOG Press, London

Steer P J 1987 Is fetal blood sampling and pH estimation helpful or harmful? Arch Dis Child 62: 1097–1098

Steer P J, Danielian P J 1994 Fetal distress in labour. In: James D K, Steer P J, Wiener C P et al (eds) High Risk Pregnancy. W B Saunders, London, pp 1077–1100

Steer P J, Eigbe F, Lissauer T J et al 1989 Interrelationships among abnormal cardiotocograms in labor, meconium staining of the amniotic fluid, arterial cord blood H, and Apgar scores. Obstet Gynecol 74: 715–721

Sykes G S, Molloy P M, Johnson P et al 1983 Fetal distress and the condition of newborn infants. Br Med J 287: 943–945

Tejani N, Mann L I, Bhakthavathsalan A et al 1975 Correlation of fetal heart rate-uterine contraction patterns with fetal scalp blood pH. Obstet Gynecol 46: 392–396

Westgate J, Harris M, Curnow J S H et al 1992 Randomised trial of cardiotocography alone or with ST waveform analysis for intrapartum monitoring. Lancet 340: 194–198

Wood C, Ng K H, Hounslow D et al 1973 Time – an important variable in normal delivery. J Obstet Gynaecol Br Cmmwlth 80: 295–300

5

Thromboembolic disease during pregnancy: A practical guide for obstetricians

J. G. Ray   J. S. Ginsberg

Thromboembolic disease (TED) during pregnancy is of major clinical importance to the obstetrician. Although deep vein thrombosis (DVT) is rare among pregnant women, with an estimated incidence ranging from 0.1–0.7 cases per 1000 pregnancies (Bergqvist et al 1983, Kierkegaard 1983), pulmonary embolism (PE) follows hypertensive diseases as the second leading cause of maternal mortality in Canada, the United States, England and Wales (Steinberg & Farine 1985; Kaunitz et al 1985; DHSS 1986). Moreover, proper treatment of patients with TED reduces the morbidity and mortality markedly (Tawes et al 1982).

This chapter covers the subject of thromboembolism in the pregnant woman. Emphasis is placed on the clinically relevant aspects of diagnosis of DVT and PE, and, in addition, the safety of maternal anticoagulant therapy for both mother and fetus is discussed at length. Finally, the management of pregnant women with valvular heart disease is discussed.

PATHOPHYSIOLOGY OF VENOUS THROMBOEMBOLISM (VTE) DURING PREGNANCY

There are several explanations why pregnancy might increase the risk of DVT formation. First, external venous compression by the gravid uterus and the engaged fetal head leads to venous stasis. In particular, the preponderance for DVT in the left leg is thought to occur as a result of compression of the left internal iliac vein by the right iliac artery (Bergqvist et al 1983; Hull et al 1990; Ginsberg et al 1991). This may also explain the higher incidence of isolated iliac vein thrombosis during pregnancy (Bergqvist et al 1983). Diminished venomotor tone from the effects of elevated progestin levels also contributes to stasis. Hypercoagulability arises secondary to increased levels of clotting factors I, II, VII, VIII, IX and X, as well as a decrease in plasma fibrinolytic activity. Hence, the increased risk of gestational DVT emerges from a milieu of stasis, and hypercoagulability.

There appears to be a relatively equal distribution for DVT among all three trimesters (24%, 47%, and 29%, respectively), noting a somewhat higher incidence during the second trimester (Bergqvist et al 1983; Ginsberg et al 1991).

DIAGNOSING VTE

Deep vein thrombosis

Thrombus in the proximal deep venous system of the thigh or pelvis – the popliteal, superficial femoral and iliac veins, or even the inferior vena cava – has a high probability of major embolization to the lungs, and patients with such disease should be treated. Calf-vein thrombosis denotes the presence of clot distal to the popliteal venous trifurcation, and poses a negligible risk of embolization provided it remains confined to the calf (Moser & LeMoine 1981). However, in non-pregnant patients, approximately 30% of calf vein thrombi extend into the proximal veins within 2 weeks of presentation and, therefore, must be identified and treated (Hall et al 1985).

Clinical suspicion of DVT

The clinician is alerted to the possibility of leg DVT when a pregnant woman presents with persistent leg swelling and/or leg pain, with tenderness upon palpation. Since non-thrombotic leg swelling is common in pregnancy, however, these symptoms and signs are non-specific. Physical examination helps to explore other processes potentially confused with DVT: ruptured Baker's cyst, muscle strain or haematoma, myositis, neurogenic pain, arthritis, bone disease, lymphangitis, and varicose veins (Weiner 1985).

As alluded to above, several studies have demonstrated a higher tendency for DVT in the left leg throughout pregnancy. In a prospective study by Ginsberg et al (1991) of 60 consecutive gravidas with documented gestational DVT, 58 were isolated to the left leg and two were bilateral. The presence of clinical signs or symptoms of clot in the left leg in a pregnant woman appears to be a sensitive clinical marker for the presence of DVT. However, if signs or symptoms are isolated to the right leg, the probability of DVT is reduced, but by no means excluded.

Venography and DVT

Contrast venography is the 'gold standard' for the diagnosis of DVT. Complete visualization of the calf, thigh and external iliac veins is possible. The adverse effects of venography include the pain associated with the examination, and the risks associated with contrast, including allergic reactions and nephrotoxicity. As Table 5.1 indicates, by applying lead-apron abdominal and pelvic shielding to the pregnant patient, the calf, popliteal and superficial femoral vein can be examined while the radiation exposure

Table 5.1   Fetal radiation exposure from various techniques used in the diagnosis of DVT and PE

Technique	Estimated fetal radiation exposure (rads)
Bilateral venography (without shielding)	0.628
Unilateral venography (without shielding)	0.314
Venography (with pelvic shielding)	< 0.050
Pulmonary angiography via femoral route	0.221–0.374
Pulmonary angiography via brachial route	< 0.050
Perfusion lung scan	0.0060–0.018
Ventilation lung scan	0.001–0.035
[125]I fibrinogen leg scanning	2.000
Plain chest X-ray	0.001

Based upon Ginsberg et al (1989).

is negligible (Ginsberg et al 1989). However, such shielding reduces visualization of the iliac vein and will not detect isolated iliac vein thrombus. In addition to the safety issues surrounding venography, it is more expensive than other non-invasive tests.

Impedance plethysmography and DVT

Impedance plethysmography (IPG) is an inexpensive, non-invasive bedside test for DVT that is sensitive to obstruction of venous outflow, as occurs with DVT. In a randomized controlled trial involving 645 non-pregnant patients with clinically suspected DVT, serial non-invasive IPG was shown to be highly effective at testing for the presence or development of proximal venous clots (Hull et al 1985). Similar results were obtained from a community hospital outpatient cohort study (Huisman et al 1989). These studies indicate that, because of its very high sensitivity, serially negative IPG essentially rules out the presence of clinically important DVT.

In addition, Hull et al (1990), performed a prospective study using serial IPG on 152 consecutive pregnant women with clinically suspected DVT. They reported that, among those 139 women with normal serial IPG, anticoagulants could be withheld safely.

For women being evaluated with IPG in the second and third trimesters, it is appropriate for them to lie in the lateral decubitus position for 20 minutes before testing to avoid compression of the deep veins by the gravid uterus and fetal head. This reduces the false-positive rate (Hull et al 1990).

Ultrasonography and DVT

The availability of real-time B-mode compression ultrasonography and Doppler flow technology has enabled non-invasive imaging for DVT to be carried a step further. Not only can ultrasound aid in the diagnosis of proximal DVT, but it is also helpful at identifying other causes of leg swelling, such as a muscle haematoma or Baker's cyst.

Prospective studies clearly support the use of B-mode ultrasonography for diagnosing DVT in non-pregnant patients (Dauzat et al 1986; Monreal et al 1989). Unlike IPG, however, ultrasonography cannot accurately rule out isolated iliac DVT, due to technical limitations (Comerota et al 1993). Prospective studies on the use of ultrasound on pregnant women with suspected DVT are pending.

Diagnosis of DVT: summary

Although there is high-quality evidence that ultrasound is better than IPG in non-pregnant subjects (Heijboer et al 1993), ultrasonography has not been validated in pregnant patients. However, it is our belief that either test is reasonable in pregnant women with suspected DVT, provided the limitations of each are understood. Regardless of which investigation is chosen, at a minimum, repeat testing should be performed in patients whose initial test is negative. Other practical issues exist. First, what is the local availability of either tests at one's facility? Second, what are the comparative skills of the ultrasonographer versus the IPG technician, since the

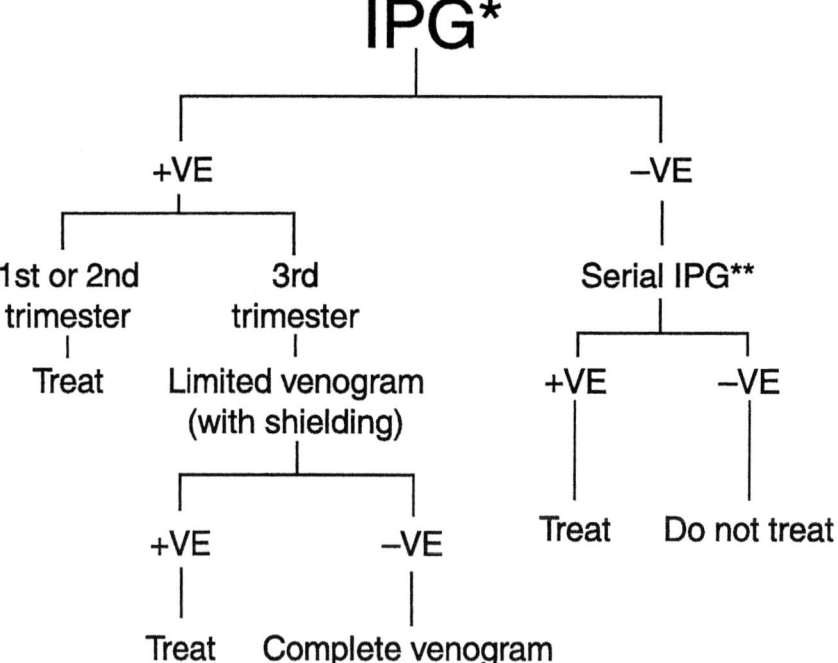

Fig. 5.1   Diagnosis of clinically suspected DVT during pregnancy using impedance plethysmography (IPG). *Women tested with IPG in the second or third trimester of pregnancy should lie in the lateral decubitus position for 20 minutes before and during the test. **IPG should be repeated on days 2, 5, 7, and between days 10 and 14.

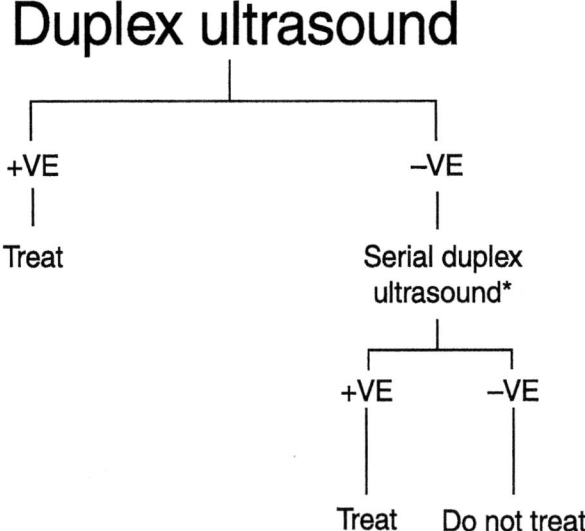

Fig. 5.2 Diagnosis of clinically suspected DVT during pregnancy using duplex ultrasonography. *Duplex ultrasound should be repeated on days 2 and 7.

accuracy of both depends upon the users' training and experience? Figure 5.1 summarizes one diagnostic approach to DVT using IPG, while Figure 5.2 outlines another approach using ultrasonography.

PULMONARY EMBOLISM (PE)

Clinical suspicion of PE

Sudden-onset dyspnea, tachypnea, or pleuritic chest pain in a gravida raises the possibility of PE. Hypotension with evidence of raised jugular venous pressure and hypoxia are quite rare, but certainly heighten one's diagnostic suspicion. Overall, however, the clinical diagnosis of PE is not reliable enough to direct decisions about therapy (Dalen 1991). Although a plain chest radiograph cannot be used to diagnose or rule out PE, it is useful in excluding other disease processes, and interpreting the ventilation/perfusion (V/Q) lung scan (Worsley et al 1993).

Diagnostic testing for PE

Pulmonary angiography is the 'gold standard' for the diagnosis of PE (Goodman 1984). The downside to this technique is its invasiveness, the associated reactions to intravenous contrast agent (Perrier et al 1994), the relatively high levels of radiation exposure (Table 5.1), and the expense. If pulmonary angiography is required, then brachial vein cannulation, combined with abdominal and pelvic lead shielding can help to minimize radiation exposure to the fetus.

Because of the limitations of pulmonary angiography, the V/Q lung scan is the pivotal test for diagnosing PE. A prospective study of 515 non-pregnant patients with suspected PE clearly demonstrated that a normal V/Q scan had very high negative predictive value for PE, and that withholding treatment in such cases was safe (Hull et al 1990).

Likewise, a 'high-probability' lung scan, as defined by a segmental or large subsegmental perfusion defect with normal ventilation, strongly supports the diagnosis of PE (PIOPED Investigators 1990). It is unclear if, and how, the pregnant state might modify these results, since prospective studies of PE during pregnancy are limited.

A common diagnostic dilemma surrounding PE is what to do if the V/Q scan is 'non-high probability' (sometimes also called 'intermediate probability', 'indeterminate' or 'inconclusive'), because patients with such lung scans have an intermediate probability (10–40%) of PE. This scenario represents approximately 50% of non-pregnant patients with suspected PE (PIOPED Investigators 1990). Of course, one may go on to perform pulmonary angiography, but again there are the associated risks as outlined above. Other clinical strategies have been developed in an attempt to resolve this issue 'less invasively'. Ultrasonography or IPG is useful in pregnant patients with a 'non-high probability' lung scan because a positive test result provides sufficient grounds for initiating anticoagulation. However, in patients with normal IPG or ultrasound, strong consideration should be given to performing pulmonary angiography since normal IPG or ultrasound cannot reliably exclude PE (Perrier et al 1994).

Diagnosis of PE: summary

Figure 5.3 provides an outline for the diagnosis of PE. A high-probability or normal lung scan essentially rules in or rules out PE, respectively. A non-high probability scan should be followed by IPG or duplex ultrasonography; if the results are positive, anticoagulants can be started, whereas, if they are negative, pulmonary angiography should be considered.

TREATMENT OF PATIENTS WITH VTE

Heparin

In non-pregnant patients, heparin has been used effectively and safely for the treatment of TED via both the intravenous and subcutaneous routes. Heparin has also been studied prospectively among several hundred pregnant women being treated for TED. It does not cross the placenta or into breast milk, nor does the evidence suggest that there are any adverse fetal

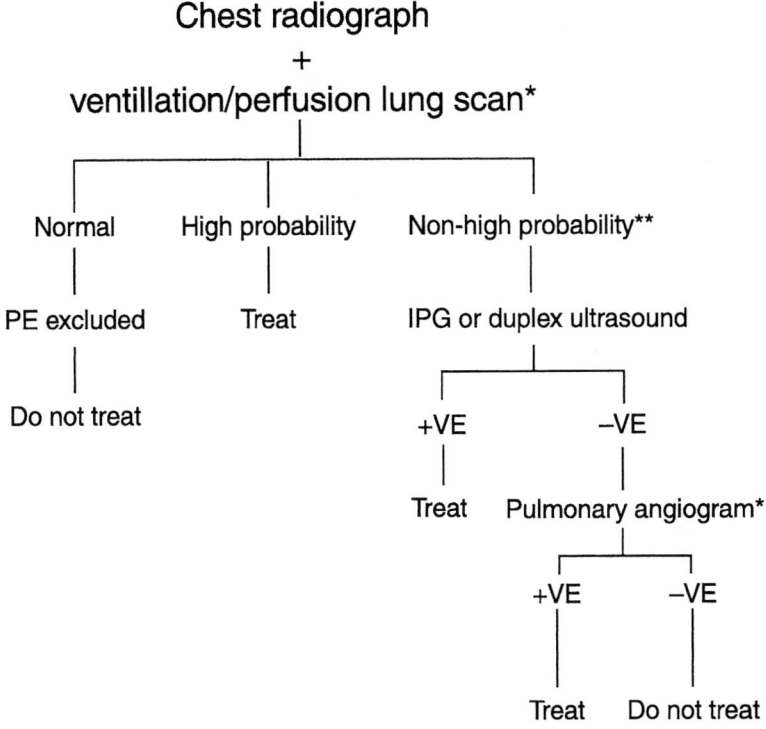

Fig. 5.3 Diagnosis of clinically suspected PE during pregnancy. *Abdominal and pelvic shielding with a lead apron is suggested. **A 'non-high probability' V/Q scan is sometimes called 'intermediate probability', 'indeterminate' or 'inconclusive'.

effects with its use (Ginsberg & Hirsh 1992). Long-term administration of heparin has been associated with loss of trabecular bone density and, rarely, osteoporotic fractures (Ginsberg et al 1990).

The current recommendation for treatment of VTE in the pregnant woman is full-dose intravenous heparin for 5–10 days, with a therapeutic endpoint of an activated partial thromboplastin time (APTT) approximately twice control. Full-dose subcutaneous heparin (to achieve APTT twice control) is then begun for the remainder of the pregnancy, and should be discontinued approximately 24 hours before elective induction of labour. In high-risk patients, intravenous heparin can be resumed, and stopped about 4–6 hours prior to the anticipated time of delivery (Anderson et al 1991). If the onset of labour is sudden, then the effect of heparin can be reversed using intravenous protamine sulphate. Immediately post-partum, full-dose subcutaneous or intravenous heparin should be begun. Warfarin should be initiated within 24 hours of delivery and once a therapeutic International Normalized Ratio (INR, formerly prothrombin time) of 2.0–3.0 is achieved, the heparin is discontinued, and the warfarin is maintained for at least 2 weeks postpartum (Ginsberg & Hirsh 1992).

Warfarin

When warfarin (coumarin) is administered during the embryonic and fetal periods, especially during the first 6–12 weeks, it is believed to be teratogenic (Iturbe-Alessio et al 1986). The warfarin molecule crosses the placenta, and is thought to cause the syndrome of warfarin embryopathy, whose manifestations include mid-face and nasal hypoplasia, optic atrophy, digital hypoplasia, stippled epiphyses (chondrodysplasia punctata), and mental retardation (Holzgreve et al 1976, Stevenson et al 1980, Iturbe-Alessio 1986).

Previous case reviews and case-control studies have challenged whether warfarin is more harmful to the fetus than heparin (Hall et al 1980; Chong et al 1984). The quality of this evidence is too poor, however, to reliably demonstrate warfarin's safety during the first trimester. While the 'jury is still out', the administration of warfarin during pregnancy cannot be endorsed at the present time. Warfarin and breast-feeding appears to be safe, however, with no detectable drug levels or anticoagulant effects on the infant with long-term administration (Ginsberg & Hirsh 1992).

Alternatives to anticoagulation

In patients with TED for whom anticoagulation is strictly contraindicated, such as intracranial haemorrhage or active bleeding, insertion of an inferior vena cava filter is a sensible alternative. The purpose of this filter is to prevent the transmission of large venous emboli to the pulmonary circulation. Although experience with such devices among pregnant patients is quite limited, relayed largely by small case series, it appears to be safe for both mother and fetus (Narayan et al 1992).

PRIOR VTE AND PREGNANCY

Among pregnant women with a history of a previous DVT or PE, and no thrombophilic state (deficiency of protein C, protein S, or antithrombin III, resistance to activated protein C or the persistent presence of antiphospholipid antibodies) the true risk of recurrent VTE is unknown, but has been estimated at 4–12% (Ginsberg & Hirsh 1992). There are presently two major options for management. The first is to administer prophylactic subcutaneous heparin at a dose of between 5000–10 000 IU twice daily (Howell et al 1983). The APTT does not need to be monitored at these doses.

The major disadvantages of long-term heparin prophylaxis include the major inconvenience of subcutaneous dosing, the risk of heparin-induced thrombocytopenia, and densitometry-proven subclinical osteoporosis (Dahlman et al 1994; Barbour et al 1994). The introduction of subcutaneous low-molecular-weight heparin (LMWH) for thromboprophylaxis may lessen these risks, and is currently raising interest as an alternative to heparin for recurrent VTE, albeit it remains very expensive at present (Gillis et al 1992, Nelson-Piercy 1994, Sturridge et al 1994).

The second option in the management of a gravida with prior VTE is to withhold prophylaxis and use clinical vigilance by the patient combined with surveillance using periodic IPG or leg ultrasonography. The goal to is monitor for the development of proximal leg DVT.

So which option is 'better'? The answer is, 'it depends'. Following the route of surveillance depends on the local availability of non-invasive testing and the reliability of the patient. If IPG or ultrasonography is possible, then it is necessary to sit down with the patient and present the pros and cons of either choice. Ultimately, if the patient is properly informed, then the decision is hers to make.

The real issue for researchers is to measure the true risk of recurrence of potentially fatal VTE in pregnancy. A randomized controlled trial comparing prophylaxis to surveillance might better answer this question, as well as which option is more prudent.

Most women with thrombophilic states and previous VTE will be receiving long-term warfarin therapy. When such women become pregnant, full-dose subcutaneous heparin should be substituted for warfarin. The management of pregnant women with thrombophilic states and no previous VTE is problematic because of the lack of clinical trials, but prophylactic doses of heparin or surveillance (as described above) would seem reasonable.

PREGNANT WOMEN WITH VALVULAR HEART DISEASE

With a rise in the number of women receiving prosthetic heart valves, there is growing concern about the management of these patients during pregnancy. Unfortunately, there is a paucity of data on this subject, and controlled clinical trials have not been done. Although mechanical heart valves last much longer than tissue valves, the former also carry a much higher risk of embolization (Ben-Ismail et al 1986), thereby necessitating thromboprophylaxis (Edmunds 1982). Those with bioprosthetic valves do not require anticoagulants, unless there is associated atrial fibrillation (Born et al 1992). A prospective study of 72 pregnancies among 63 women with either tissue or mechanical heart valves determined that warfarin exposure during the first 6–12 weeks of gestation was unsafe for the fetus, due to high rates of teratogenicity (25%) and spontaneous abortion (16.2%) (Iturbe-Alessio et al 1986). Among those women with mechanical valves, or bioprosthetic valves and atrial fibrillation, the data support the safe and efficacious use of therapeutic warfarin (INR greater than two) after the 12th week of pregnancy, until 2 weeks prior to delivery. Before the 12th and after the 36–37th weeks of pregnancy, it seems reasonable to administer a therapeutic dose of subcutaneous heparin (e.g. 17 500 U every 12 hours) for a target mid-dosing APTT of at least twice control, to be followed with judicious monitoring. This switch to heparin lessens the likelihood of teratogenicity and fetal haemorrhage associated with early and late warfarin use, respectively. Lower doses of heparin (e.g. 5000 U every 12 hours) do not appear to provide adequate protection against thromboembolic complications (Caruso et al 1994).

An alternative approach to warfarin and heparin is to administer a therapeutic dose of subcutaneous heparin (mid-dosing APTT of at least twice control) throughout the pregnancy. This eliminates the small risk of central nervous system and optic tract abnormalities described with warfarin exposure even after the first trimester. Again, a decision is made by the patient after she has been properly informed of the advantages and disadvantages of each option.

The addition of low-dose aspirin (80–100 mg once daily) to warfarin prophylaxis among non-pregnant patients with mechanical heart valves has been shown to lower the rate of embolic stroke without increasing haemorrhagic complications (Turpie et al 1993). The safety of low-dose aspirin during pregnancy has been well demonstrated in several randomized controlled trials of pregnancy-induced hypertension and pre-eclampsia. Although there is little direct evidence available to support its benefit in pregnant patients, we endorse the addition of low-dose aspirin to anticoagulants among pregnant women with mechanical valves because of the strength of the data and potential benefits in the non-pregnant population. Any woman of childbearing age who requires valvular surgery, or who is presently taking warfarin, needs to be informed about the risks associated with warfarin use during pregnancy, as well as the effects of pregnancy and delivery on cardiac function. Proper contraception, and careful planning and testing for pregnancy, can enable most women with prosthetic cardiac valves to carry a child to term while reducing the risk of harm to herself and her fetus.

FUTURE CONSIDERATIONS IN VTE

D-dimer is a fibrin degradation product that can be quantified in plasma using enzyme-linked immunosorbent assays (ELISA), latex agglutination, and whole-blood red-cell agglutination assays. Recent prospective data (Goldhaber et al 1993; Ginsberg et al 1995) suggest that a low D-dimer blood level excludes PE. Studies of pregnant women will likely be done as the test gains acceptance in the general population.

In terms of new modalities for the treatment of VTE, the development of LMWH offers a promising alternative in the treatment of patients with VTE. The drug's pharmacokinetic behaviour is more predictable than LMWH, with a more direct relationship between dose and response. Fewer adverse effects, such as haemorrhage, heparin-induced thrombocytopenia, or osteoporosis seem to arise with LMWH (Nelson-Piercy 1994). It is also more convenient because of its possible once-daily dosing.

LMWH does not appear to cross the placenta and is therefore safe during pregnancy (Forestier et al 1984; Melissari et al 1992). In a study by Melissari et al (1992), using LMWH in 11 pregnancies complicated by VTE, there were no demonstrable adverse outcomes to mother or child. Future controlled studies will likely prove that LMWH is safer and more efficacious during pregnancy. Until that time, heparin remains the drug of choice unless specific contraindications to its use arise.

KEY POINTS FOR CLINICAL PRACTICE

1. Clinical diagnosis of venous thrombosis and pulmomary embolism is unreliable necessitating accurate objective tests.

2. For patients with suspected deep vein thrombosis, we recommend serial IPG or ultrasonography.

3. In patients with suspected pulmonary embolism, ventilation/perfusion lung scanning should be the initial test performed during any stage of pregnancy.

4. Heparin is the anticoagulant of choice during pregnancy and the use of warfarin should be restricted to the second and early third trimesters if necessary.

5. In women with acute venous thromboembolism during pregnancy, full-dose intravenous heparin followed by adjusted dose subcutaneous heparin should be used.

6. In pregnant women with prior venous thromboembolism, either low dose heparin therapy throughout pregnancy or clinical vigilance combined with non-invasive testing should be considered.

7. In pregnant women with valvular heart disease, high doses of subcutaneous heparin should be used either throughout pregnancy or in combination with warfarin whereby heparin is used during the first trimester, warfarin during the second and early third trimesters and heparin prior to delivery. The addition of low-dose aspirin to either regimen seems reasonable.

REFERENCES

Anderson D R, Ginsberg J S, Burrows R et al 1991 Subcutaneous heparin therapy during pregnancy: a need for concern at the time of delivery. Thromb Haemost 65: 248–250

Barbour L A, Kick S D, Steiner J F et al 1994 A prospective study of heparin-induced osteoporosis in pregnancy using bone densitometry. Am J Obstet Gynecol 170: 862–869

Ben-Ismail M, Abid F, Trabelsi S et al 1986 Cardiac valve prostheses, anticoagulation and pregnancy. Br Heart J 55: 101–105

Bergqvist A, Bergqvist D, Hallbook T 1983 Deep vein thrombosis during pregnancy: a prospective study. Acta Obstet Gynecol Scand 62: 443–448

Born D, Martinez E E, Almeida P A M et al 1992 Pregnancy in patients with prosthetic heart valves: the effects of anticoagulation on mother, fetus, and neonate. Am Heart J 124: 413–417

Caruso A C, Carolis S D, Ferrazzani S 1994 Pregnancy outcome in women with cardiac valve prosthesis. Eur J Obstet Gynecol 54: 7–11

Chong M K B, Harvey D, de Swiet M 1984 Follow-up study of children whose mothers were treated with warfarin during pregnancy. Br J Obstet Gynaecol 91: 1070–1073

Comerota A J, Katz M L, Hashemi H A 1993 Venous duplex imaging for the diagnosis of acute deep venous thrombosis. Haemostasis 23 (suppl 1): 61–71

DHSS 1986 Report on confidential inquiries into maternal deaths for England and Wales 1979–1981. HMSO, London

Dahlman T C, Sjoberg H E, Ringertz H 1994 Bone mineral density during long-term prophylaxis with heparin in pregnancy. Am J Obstet Gynecol 170: 1315–1320

Dalen J E 1991 Clinical diagnosis of acute pulmonary embolism: when should a V/Q scan be ordered? Chest 100: 1185–1186

Dauzat M M, Laroche J P, Charras C et al 1986 Real-time B-mode ultrasonography for better specificity in the non-invasive diagnosis of deep vein thrombosis. J Ultrasound Med 5: 625–631

Edmunds Jr L H 1982 Thromboembolic complications of current cardiac valvular prostheses. Ann Thorac Surg 34: 96–106

Forestier F, Daffos E, Cappella-Pavlovsky M 1984 Low molecular weight heparin (PK 10169) does not cross the placenta during the second trimester of pregnancy: study by direct fetal blood sampling under ultrasound. Thromb Res 34: 557–560

Gillis S, Shushan A, Eldor A 1992 Use of low molecular weight heparin for prophylaxis and treatment of thromboembolism in pregnancy. Int J Gynecol Obstet 39: 297–301

Ginsberg J S, Hirsh J 1992 Use of antithrombotic agents during pregnancy. Chest 102 (Suppl): 385S–390S

Ginsberg S, Hirsh J, Rainbow A J et al 1989 Risks to the fetus of radiologic procedures used in the diagnosis of maternal venous thromboembolic disease. Thromb Haemost 61: 189–196

Ginsberg J S, Kowalchuk G, Hirsh J et al 1990 Heparin effect on bone density. Thromb Haemost 64: 286–289

Ginsberg J S, Brill-Edwards P, Bona R et al 1991 Deep vein thrombosis (DVT) during pregnancy: leg and trimester of presentation. Thromb Haemost 65: 720a

Ginsberg J S, Wells P S, Brill-Edwards P et al 1995 Application of a novel and rapid whole blood assay for D-dimer in patients with clinically suspected pulmonary embolism. Thromb Haemost 73: 35–38

Goldhaber S Z, Simons G R, Eliott C G et al 1993 Quantitative plasma D-dimer levels among patients undergoing pulmonary angiography for suspected pulmonary embolism. JAMA 270: 2819–2822

Goodman P C 1984 Pulmonary angiography Clin Chest Med 5: 465–477

Hall J G, Pauli R M, Wilson K M 1980 Maternal and fetal sequelae of anticoagulation during pregnancy. Am J Med 68: 122–140

Heijboer H, Buller H R, Lensing A W A et al 1993 A comparison of real-time compression ultrasonography with impedance plethysmography for the diagnosis of deep-vein thrombosis in symptomatic outpatients. N Engl J Med 329: 1365–1369

Holzgreve W, Carey J C, Hall B D 1976 Warfarin-induced fetal abnormalities. Lancet ii: 194–195

Howell R, Fidler J, Letsky E et al 1983 The risks of antenatal subcutaneous heparin prophylaxis: a controlled trial. Br J Obstet Gynecol 90: 1124–1128

Huisman M V, Buller H R, ten Cate J W et al 1989 Management of clinically suspected acute venous thrombosis in outpatients with serial impedance plethysmography in a community hospital setting. Arch Intern Med 149: 511–513

Hull R D, Hirsh J, Carter C J et al 1985 Diagnostic efficacy of impedance plethysmography for clinically suspected deep-vein thrombosis. Ann Intern Med 102: 21–28

Hull R D, Raskob G E, Carter C J 1990a Serial impedance plethysmography in pregnant patients with clinically suspected deep-vein thrombosis: clinical validity of negative findings. Ann Intern Med 112: 663–667

Hull R D, Raskob G E, Coates G et al 1990b Clinical validity of a normal perfusion lung scan in patients with suspected pulmonary embolism. Chest 97: 23–26

Iturbe-Alessio I, del Carmen Fonseca M, Mutchinik O et al 1986 Risks of anticoagulant therapy in pregnant women with artificial heart valves. N Engl J Med 315: 1390–1393

Kaunitz A M, Hughes J M, Grimes D A et al 1985 Causes of maternal mortality in the United States. Obstet Gynecol 65: 605–612

Kierkegaard A 1983 Incidence and diagnosis of deep vein thrombosis associated with pregnancy. Acta Obstet Gynecol Scand 62: 239–243

Many A, Pauzner R, Carp H et al 1992 Treatment of patients with antiphospholipid antibodies during pregnancy. Am J Reprod Immunol 28: 216–218

Melissari E, Parker C, Wilson N V et al 1992 Use of low molecular weight heparin in pregnancy. Thromb Haemost 68: 652–656

Monreal M, Montserrat E, Salvador R et al 1989 Real-time ultrasound for diagnosis of symptomatic venous thrombosis and for screening patients at risk: correlation with ascending conventional venography. Angiology 40: 527–533

Mosely P, Kerstein M D 1980 Pregnancy and thrombophlebitis. Surg Gynecol Obstet 150: 593–599

Moser K, LeMoine J 1981 Is embolic risk conditioned by location of deep venous thrombosis? Ann Intern Med 94: 439–444

Narayan H, Krarup K, Thurston H et al 1992 Experience with the Cardial inferior vena cava filter as prophylaxis against pulmonary embolism in pregnant women with extensive deep venous thrombosis. Br J Obstet Gynaecol 99: 637–640

Nelson-Piercy C 1994 Low molecular weight heparin for obstetric thromboprophylaxis. Br J Obstet Gynaecol 101: 6–8

Out H J, Bruinse H W, Godelieve C M L et al 1992 A prospective, controlled multicenter study on the obstetric risks of pregnant women with antiphospholipid antibodies. Am J Obstet Gynecol 167: 26–32

Perrier A, Bounameaux H, Morabia A et al 1994 Contribution of D-dimer plasma measurement and lower-limb venous ultrasound to the diagnosis of pulmonary embolism: a decision analysis model. Am Heart J 127: 624–635

PIOPED Investigators 1990 Value of the ventilation/perfusion scan in acute pulmonary embolism. Results of the prospective investigation of pulmonary embolism diagnosis (PIOPED). JAMA 263: 2753–2759

Silver R M, Draper M L, Scott J R et al 1994 Clinical consequences of antiphospholipid antibodies: an historical cohort study. Obstet Gynecol 83: 372–377

Steinberg W M, Farine D 1985 Maternal mortality in Ontario from 1970 to 1980. Obstet Gynecol 66: 510–512

Stevenson R E, Burton O M, Ferlauto G J, Taylor H A 1980 Hazards of oral anticoagulation during pregnancy. JAMA 243: 1549–1551

Tawes R L, Kennedy P A, Harris E J et al 1982 Management of deep venous thrombosis and pulmonary embolism during pregnancy. Am J Surg 144: 141–145

Turpie A G G, Gent M, Laupacis A 1993 A comparison of aspirin with placebo in patients treated with warfarin after heart valve replacement. N Engl J Med 329: 524–529

Sturridge F, de Swiet M, Letsky E 1994 The use of low molecular weight heparin for thromboprophylaxis in pregnancy. Br J Obstet Gynaecol 101: 69–71

Weiner C P 1985 Diagnosis and management of thromboembolic disease during pregnancy. Clin Obstet Gynecol 28: 107–118

Worsley D F, Alavi A, Aronchick et al 1993 Chest radiographic findings in patients with acute pulmonary embolism: observations from the PIOPED study. Radiology 189: 133–136

6

Malignant disease and pregnancy

D. N. Carney

Cancer is a leading cause of death among women of childbearing age. However, cancer occurring in a pregnant patient is a rare event, with a reported incidence of 0.1%-0.7% (Allen & Nisker 1986; Doll et al 1988; Jones et al 1991). It is also estimated that pregnant women with cancer account for nearly 0.8% of all cancer cases in women. In the US almost 3500 cases of cancer occur in pregnant women annually, about 1 in 1000 pregnancies. Because of the younger age of childbearing women, the cancers most frequently observed are those usually seen in this age group, namely, malignant lymphomas, Hodgkin's disease, leukaemias, breast cancer, melanoma, and cancers of the cervix, thyroid and colon. The marked rise of lung cancer in young women recorded recently suggests that this cancer will become more frequently observed in pregnant women in the years ahead. No evidence exists of an increased incidence of cancer in pregnant patients compared with the control population. In addition, no convincing data suggests that pregnancy itself adversely affects either the prognosis or the biology of the maternal cancer (Jones et al 1991).

The diagnosis of cancer in pregnancy poses a range of problems. For the mother the immediate fear is that not only may she die from her disease, but also that she may lose her child. She may believe that because of her pregnancy appropriate treatment for her cancer could be withheld. For the physician caring for the patient, the diagnosis of cancer in pregnancy raises many issues including psychosocial, ethical, medical, religious, ethnic, etc. Thus the need for individualized treatment must be stressed. The decisions regarding the treatment of a pregnant patient with cancer can best be achieved through a multi-disciplinary approach involving the patient's obstetrician, family physician, oncologist, paediatrician and neonatologist, as well as the patient and her family, the supporting medical staff and the clergy. The medical team together can provide for the best outcome, namely a healthy mother and child. While the team approach is essential, one member, e.g. the oncologist, should act as a spokesperson when communicating with the mother and family.

This review will focus on the use of chemotherapy in the pregnant patient, and the management of specific cancers that may arise in the pregnant patient.

CHEMOTHERAPY IN PREGNANCY

In the consideration of the use of chemotherapy in pregnancy two factors must be considered: 1) the pharmacology of the agents and 2) the immediate and delayed effects of the cytotoxic agents on the developing fetus (Beeley 1986; Doll et al 1989; Doll 1992).

The pharmacology of cytotoxic agents during pregnancy

Many of the physiological changes associated with pregnancy may alter the pharmacokinetics of cytotoxic agents. Delayed gastric emptying and gastrointestinal motility may alter the rate and degree of drug absorption. The expanded plasma volume and increase in total body water of approximately 50% may, by a dilutional effect, reduce peak drug concentration. In addition, the half-life may also be prolonged. The resulting alteration in the 'concentration x time' relationship of cytotoxic agents may therefore result in an alteration of therapeutic efficacy and lead to enhanced toxicity. In pregnancy, albumin concentration decreases and plasma proteins increase since many cytotoxic agents compete for binding sites on albumin and other plasma proteins. Such changes may affect drug distribution and plasma concentration. The amniotic fluid may function as a pharmacological third space; if so this could have major therapeutic implications with agents such as methotrexate where such 'third space' (e.g. pleural effusion) delays drug elimination and leads to increased toxicity. Finally, other changes including altered rate of hepatic oxidation, increased renal plasma flow, glomerular filtration rate and creatinine clearance may also alter the pharmacokinetics of administered cytotoxic agents. While the above changes exist in the pregnant women, their impact on the outcome when chemotherapy is used remains unclear. In the absence of hard data it should be assumed that the drug dosage in the pregnant state should mimic that used in the non-pregnant state. However, close monitoring of the patient because of altered toxicity and efficacy is necessary.

A number of factors may also influence transplacental drug delivery (Doll 1992). The placenta is the portal of entry for drugs to the fetus. Factors favouring transplacental transport include drugs with a low-molecular weight, high lipid solubility, non-ionization and loose binding to plasma proteins. As most chemotherapeutic agents possess these characteristics, the majority readily enter the fetal circulation.

Within the fetus the immature liver may metabolize drugs by oxidation while the fetal kidneys may be involved in drug elimination. Drugs which are excreted into the amniotic fluid may be ingested by the fetus and absorbed from the gastrointestinal tract, thereby increasing exposure of the fetus to these cytotoxic agents and potentially increasing any cytotoxic effects to the fetus.

Finally, as the placenta is the major route of drug excretion from the fetus, the administration of cytotoxic agents shortly before birth may cause unpredictable fetal toxicity because of the delayed metabolism and excretion in the neonate when placental excretion can no longer occur.

The effects of cytotoxic agents on the fetus and neonate (Table 6.1)

The impact of cytotoxic agents on the developing fetus is directly related to the timing of such exposure. The embryonic period of fetal development commences during the third week after ovulation (Jones et al 1991). Over the next 6 weeks the embryo grows in length and all major organs are formed. This embryonic period ends and the fetal period begins 8 weeks after ovulation and corresponds to a gestational age of 10 weeks. During the fetal period the growth and maturation of the newly formed structures takes place. The greatest risk in the developing fetus to cytotoxic agents is therefore during the embryonic period or first trimester. Susceptibility to cytotoxic agents decreases as organ formation advances and becomes almost negligible once organogenesis is completed.

The effects of chemotherapeutic agents on the fetus can be subdivided into immediate and delayed (Table 6.1) (Doll 1992). If administered during the first week after conception either a spontaneous abortion or no effect may be observed ('all or nothing phenomenon'). Exposure in the first trimester can cause congenital malformations and/or an abortion. During the second and third trimesters drugs rarely cause malformation. However, fetal growth and development may be impaired.

Moreover, as neuronal growth continues through this period, exposure to cytotoxic agents may cause microcephaly, mental retardation and impaired learning.

Table 6.1   Chemotherapy during pregnancy and risk of fetal malformations

	Alkylating[a] agents	Antimetabolites[b]	Antibiotics[b]	Plant[b] alkaloids	Combination[b]	Total[b]
First trimester	6/44	15/77	0/1	1/14	7/45	29/181 (16.2%)
Second and third trimester	1/26	0/38	0/1	0/6	1/79	2/150 (1.3%)

[b]No. of fetal malformations/no. exposed patients
Modified with permission from Doll et al (1989)

Teratogenesis from chemotherapeutic agents

Many factors may influence the probability of teratogenesis from anti-cancer agents. These include:

1. the timing of exposure to the cytotoxic agent
2. the cytotoxic agent used
3. the total drug dosage, the frequency of administration and duration of drug exposure
4. whether one or more chemotherapeutic agents are used in combination or sequentially, or combined modality therapy, i.e. chemotherapy and radiation therapy are used
5. individual and genetic susceptibility.

With few exceptions, fetal malformations are only noted in women exposed to cytotoxic agents and radiation therapy during the first trimester (Beeley 1986, Doll et al 1989). As noted in Table 6.1 a number of cytotoxic agents, given alone or in combination, may be teratogenetic when administered during this time period. Nevertheless, the overall incidence observed of 17% should be compared with the incidence of congenital malformations of 3% in all births, and the incidence of minor malformations which may be as high as 9%. Additionally, in many reports of malformations observed in women receiving chemotherapeutic agents, radiation therapy was also administered. Most cases of fetal malformation have been noted in women receiving either antimetabolites or alkylating agents. The folic acid antagonists aminopterin and methotrexate have been reported more frequently than any other agent to be associated with fetal abnormalities when given during the first trimester.

Antimetabolites including pyrimidines such as cytabarine or fluorouracil, antifols such as methotrexate and aminopterin, and thiopurines such as 6-thioguanine or 6-metocaptopurine comprise the most potent cancer drug teratogens (Clark & Chua 1989). A syndrome of congenital abnormalities associated with aminopterin (the aminopterin syndrome) including cranial dysostosis, hypertelorism, widening of the nasal bridge, anomalies of the external ears and micrognathia has been described. Because of the high risk of teratogenic effects the use of folic acid antagonists particularly during the first trimester should be avoided. In contrast to the antimetabolites, alkylating agents appear to be less potent teratogens.

The incidence of fetal malformations observed with combination chemotherapy is similar to that observed with single-agent treatment. Procarbazine, which is known to be highly mutagenic, and an integral part of the MOPP regimen for Hodgkin's disease, appears to be associated with a high incidence of fetal malformations. In contrast to the above, the vinca alkaloids (e.g. vincristine) and the antibiotics (e.g. doxorubicin) appear to carry little risk of teratogenicity even when used in the first trimester. While the risk of teratogenic effects with chemotherapeutic agents used alone or in combination during the first trimester may, with some agents, appear to be very low, the identification of serious adverse effects to the fetus may be delayed. For these reasons any infant exposed in utero to cytotoxic agents must have long-term follow-up.

In contrast to the first trimester there is no evidence of an increased risk of teratogenicity associated with the administration of chemotherapeutic drugs during the second and third trimesters (Table 6.1). Nevertheless in utero exposure cannot be considered entirely safe during this time as delayed adverse effects may arise. In addition to teratogenic effects, the use of chemotherapy during pregnancy may have effects on the fetus such as low birthweight, intrauterine growth retardation, spontaneous abortion, premature births, mental retardation, and major organ toxicity. Likewise the development of chemotherapy-induced side effects in the mother, e.g. septicaemia secondary to myelosuppression, may also affect the developing fetus.

THE ADMINISTRATION OF CHEMOTHERAPY DURING PREGNANCY

Chemotherapy during pregnancy has always the potential for causing harm, including death, to the developing fetus. The advantage of using these agents during pregnancy must therefore clearly outweigh the risks. Several factors must be taken into consideration before chemotherapy is administered during pregnancy.
These include:

1. The primary tumour and stage of the disease
2. The sensitivity of the tumour to systemic chemotherapy
3. The likely results of using chemotherapy at this time point, i.e. cure of the disease or palliation
4. The gestational period of the pregnancy
5. The opinions of the parents of the child.

The decision to use chemotherapy during pregnancy must be based primarily on the likely benefit to the mother. If cure is a realistic goal, and to achieve this the immediate institution of chemotherapy is essential, then therapy should be administered without delay (e.g. high grade non-Hodgkin's lymphoma). In contrast, where cure or even significant palliation is not attainable with systemic chemotherapy (e.g. metastatic malignant melanoma, non small-cell lung cancer), the primary goal should be protection of the fetus and avoidance of any substances likely to be harmful.

Chemotherapy, if possible, should be avoided during the first trimester. During the second and third trimester, as previously discussed, its use is not associated with any great risk of malformation, although as yet unrecognized adverse effects on the fetus may occur. If indicated, selective chemotherapeutic agents, which appear to be associated with a low risk to the fetus, can be safely administered during this time. For those cancers where chemotherapy has a major role in eradicating the disease there are no treatment regimens for which an alternative agent cannot be substituted. Thus the avoidance of agents such as antimetabolites, procarbazine, etc. throughout the pregnancy should be mandatory.

The use of chemotherapy in pregnancy is essentially a team decision aimed at the best possible outcome for both mother and child. The mother and family must be involved in the decision-making process and be aware of any potential risk to the developing fetus. In the pregnant patient receiving chemotherapy, close monitoring of blood counts etc. is essential to reduce the risk of essential toxicity associated with myelosuppression. Delivery of the infant should be planned when blood counts are optimal. In situations where high-dose intensive chemotherapy schedules are essential for cure, the author recommends that delivery should be planned and carried out at a time deemed safe for the developing fetus and where the likelihood of long-term survival is high, i.e. 28-32 weeks gestation. The timing is best decided in consultation with the neonatologist. This would reduce the duration of exposure of the fetus to chemotherapeutic agents.

Following delivery the fetus should be examined in detail for any congenital malformations and haematological investigations carried out. Breast feeding is contraindicated. Long-term follow-up of the child should be arranged.

Surgery in the cancer patient

Pregnancy is not a contraindication to surgical management of cancer. Of all the options for treating cancer in pregnancy surgery is the least likely to affect the pregnancy and, especially in the second and third trimester, can be performed with minimal risk to the fetus (Jones et al 1991).

Radiation therapy during pregnancy

As with chemotherapy the decision to use radiation therapy during pregnancy should consider all the issues involved i.e. effectiveness, goal, risk to fetus, gestation period, etc. The effects of radiation on the developing fetus include growth retardation, teratogenesis, and both fetal and neonatal death. The maximum fetal sensitivity is from 8-20 weeks gestation. Even extreme low-dose radiation therapy may be associated with long-term risk to the fetus. The fetal exposure to radiation includes external scatter and leakage from the radiation unit, both of which can be protected by shielding. However, with internal scatter of radiation, which varies with the field size and distance from field centre, the fetus cannot be protected. The risk to the fetus from chemotherapy can be significantly increased by the combined use of radiation therapy. Unless an emergency situation exists, the use of radiation therapy in pregnancy should be avoided (Jones et al 1991).

BREAST CANCER IN PREGNANCY

Breast cancer is the most common cancer in women of reproductive age. In pregnancy, breast cancer is rare, arising in approximately 3 per 10 000 deliveries (Petrek 1987). Overall, between 1 and 3% of all breast cancers occur in pregnancy. However, as these figures include all patients with breast cancer, irrespective of age, the incidence among breast cancer patients less than 40 years of age may be considerably higher.

The diagnosis of breast cancer in pregnancy is frequently delayed (Gallenberg & Loprinzi 1989; Parente et al 1988; Zemlickis et al 1992; Jones et al 1991; Petrek 1987). Delays in diagnosis of up to 6 months are not uncommon and may account for the more advanced stage of disease frequently noted in these patients. The normal physiological changes which occur in the breast during pregnancy including increased firmness, nodularity and hypertrophy may obscure an underlying mass. These changes may also make mammography examination difficult to interpret at this time.

In a suspicious breast lesion the approach to confirming a diagnosis of breast cancer in a pregnant patient is similar to that of non-pregnant women. Fine-needle aspirates of breast tumours, needle biopsies, and excisional biopsies are all safe procedures. Once the diagnosis is confirmed the appropriate treatment can be planned.

Staging procedures should include a detailed physical examination, chest X-ray, hepatic ultrasound and laboratory investigations. Radionuclide scans and CT scans should be avoided until after delivery. The safety of magnetic resonance imaging remains to be determined.

Pathological evaluation of breast cancer in pregnancy reveals similar tumours to that observed in the non-pregnant woman. However, in general, tumours appear to be of a more advanced stage, usually because of delayed diagnosis. The majority of cancers observed are high grade, oestrogen-receptor negative, with a high proliferative rate and a high incidence of lymph node metastases. These features account for the more aggressive behaviour of breast cancer in pregnancy rather than reflecting a direct or indirect effect of the pregnancy itself on the biology of the tumour (Petrek 1987).

Treatment planning should evolve along the lines of that of a non-pregnant female, namely, local control and eradication of systemic micrometastases. Because of the pathological features noted, and their premenopausal status, all women should be considered for adjuvant systemic chemotherapy.

Local control should be either a modified radical mastectomy with axillary sampling or, where suitable, a segmental resection. If the latter procedure is carried out then radiation therapy could be deferred until delivery has been completed. Chemotherapy should be administered to all patients (Theriault et al 1992). Unless there is evidence of metastatic disease this could be delayed until the second trimester. The choice of drugs should take into consideration the general principles of the use of chemotherapy in pregnancy including the avoidance of methotrexate. After delivery further additional staging procedures including radionuclide bone scanning can be safely performed and additional therapy including chemotherapy and radiation therapy can be completed.

For many years it was felt that the prognosis for women who developed breast cancer in pregnancy was significantly worse than in non-pregnant women. More recent data suggests that stage-for-stage the outcome for pregnant women with breast cancer is similar to that of their non-pregnant counterparts, particularly if they are managed in an identical fashion with appropriate use of surgery, radiation therapy and systemic chemotherapy (Jones et al 1991). Since pregnant women tend to have a more advanced stage, and are more likely to have a delay in detection, their long-term outlook, compared to all women with breast cancer in the same group, is poorer (Nugent et al 1985; Parente et al 1988; Petrek et al 1991; Willemse et al 1990). The fetal outcome of women with breast cancer while pregnant is excellent and not different from control populations. Long-term assessment is, however, needed to monitor for delayed adverse effects of treatment.

In a recent study Zemlickis et al (1992) evaluated the outcome of 118 women with breast cancer who were pregnant at the time of diagnosis. The results, matched for age, stage and treatment, were compared with 269 non-pregnant women. The study covered the period 1958-1987. Although various treatments were utilized (chemotherapy, radiation therapy, surgery, or a combination of these) no statistically significant difference in survival was noted between pregnant and non-pregnant women. Stage-for-stage the survival of the pregnant women was the same as that for non-pregnant women. Moreover, the timing of the diagnosis of breast cancer (first, second or third trimester) did not affect survival. In addition, the survival of women whose pregnancies were maintained to delivery was the same as that of women whose pregnancies were terminated prematurely. In general, the mean birthweight of infants born to women with cancer was significantly lower than that of women in the control group, even when the data were corrected for gestational age. This study shows that although breast cancer in pregnancy is frequently diagnosed at a more advanced stage than control women, stage-for-stage, women who develop breast cancer while pregnant have the same outcome as non-pregnant women.

Theriault et al (1992), studied 11 patients with breast cancer diagnosed during pregnancy. Four patients had Stage II disease, 5 Stage III and 2 Stage IV. All patients received chemotherapy (cyclophosphamide, adriamycin and 5 fluorouracil every 28 days) which was begun after the first trimester. Of the 10 normal deliveries, only 1 was complicated by neutropenia/respiratory distress in 1 infant. All infants survived and follow-up at 24 months revealed all infants had achieved normal milestones, and all mothers remained in remission. Thus it suggests that the proper use of adjuvant chemotherapy (avoiding methotrexate) is safe during the second and third trimesters, thereby allowing appropriate treatment for the mother with little or modest short-term risk to the infant.

The role or need for termination of pregnancy in the pregnant patient with breast cancer has to be considered (Clark & Chua 1989; Petrek 1987). In the late 1940s and 1950s termination was regarded as an integral part of the management of the breast cancer patient who was pregnant. Recent data, however, have not shown any survival advantage for women who undergo a therapeutic abortion as part of their management, irrespective of the gestation time when the diagnosis of breast cancer is made (Clark & Chua 1989). When compared with standard therapy, the benefit of routine abortion cannot be demonstrated. In the rare instance where the breast cancer is extremely aggressive and presents with metastatic disease, and appropriate therapeutic intervention cannot be carried out because of the risk to the fetus (e.g. radiation therapy for spinal cord compression), the need for termination of the pregnancy in this rare individual case should be discussed with the mother and family, and a joint decision reached. In this situation, however, the mother is unlikely to be cured of her disease, thus protection of the fetus should be a major concern.

Pregnancy following breast cancer

No data supports the view that pregnancy following a diagnosis of breast cancer adversely affects the disease process (Clark & Chua 1989). For all women who wish to have children following a diagnosis of breast cancer, a delay of at least 2 years is recommended. This would allow aggressive disease to appear. If the woman remains disease-free after 2 years, a subsequent pregnancy has not been shown to be detrimental to her health. Many studies have shown that the outcome in women who become pregnant after this time is excellent and the same, or even slightly better, than breast cancer patients with no subsequent pregnancies (Sutton et al 1990; Clarke & Chua 1989; Daly & Donnellan 1992). No data supports the need for termination of a pregnancy in patients who are disease-free following a previous diagnosis of breast carcinoma.

CERVICAL CANCER AND PREGNANCY

Cervical cancer is the most frequently diagnosed cancer in pregnancy (Jolles 1989; Perez & Brady 1992). Since the usual symptom of cervical cancer is vaginal bleeding this is often attributed to the pregnancy resulting in a delay in diagnosis. Women with cervical cancer in pregnancy more often have Stage I disease compared to non-pregnant patients. An examination of the cervix should be encouraged for all women at the first or second prenatal visit and should be routine in any women with bleeding or discharge during pregnancy. The biology of cervical cancer does not appear to be altered by pregnancy.

Treatment depends both on the stage of the disease and the gestational age (Jolles 1989). During the first trimester and first half of the second trimester, the institution of curative treatment should be carried out to avoid any unnecessary risks to the mother. Thus Stage IB and Stage IIA disease are best managed by radical hysterectomy and bilateral pelvic lymph-adenectomy. If disease is diagnosed late in the second trimester or into the third trimester consideration should be given to fetal survival. A short delay in treatment should be considered if this permits fetal viability to be attained (e.g. 28 weeks gestation) before definitive therapy is commenced. Following acceleration of lung surfactant with cortisone in the third trimester, delivery by caesarean section followed by immediate radical hysterectomy and lymph node dissection for early-stage disease, or aggressive radiation therapy for more advanced disease, should be instituted. In these patients a vaginal delivery should be avoided. The prognosis for women with cervical cancer diagnosed during pregnancy is essentially the same as that for the non-pregnant woman (Hopkins & Morley 1992).

LEUKAEMIAS AND LYMPHOMAS IN PREGNANCY

The incidence of leukaemia in pregnancy is extremely low 'approximately 1 in 100 000 pregnancies' (Sutcliffe & Chapman 1986; Catanzarite & Ferguson 1984). The majority of cases are diagnosed during routine antenatal care.

Because of the age group, the majority are cases of acute myelogenous leukaemia. No data shows that the biological behaviour of the leukaemia is altered by pregnancy.

Because of the small number of cases, treatment guidelines are difficult. Although the risk of teratogenesis is real, there are many case reports of successful combination chemotherapy administered during the first trimester resulting in complete remission and the delivery of healthy babies (Reynoso et al 1987; Pizzuto et al 1980; Dara et al 1981; Aviles & Niz 1988). The small number of congenital abnormalities noted may be directly related to the use of agents not associated with a high risk of fetal abnormalities e.g. doxorubicin. As for other tumours, avoidance of antifolates and alkylating agents during the first trimester is recommended if at all possible. The use of the antracycline antibiotics, the vinca alkaloids, the antipyrimidine cytabarine, and prednisone appear to be associated with a very low risk of fetal abnormalities and are highly potent agents for treating acute leukaemia. Fortunately, as the majority of cases are diagnosed in the third trimester, the fetal exposure to several courses of chemotherapy is minimized with delivery recommended as soon as fetal survival is assured thereby allowing the continued use of more intensive chemotherapy.

Management of intermediate and high-grade non-Hodgkin's lymphomas

(NHL) should follow similar lines to acute leukaemia, as immediate treatment is essential if a cure is to be obtained (Steiner-Salz et al 1985; Ioachim 1989; Sutcliffe & Chapman 1986; Ward & Weiss 1989). Careful selection of chemotherapeutic agents should minimize risk to the fetus.

The evaluation and management of patients diagnosed with Hodgkin's disease during pregnancy is somewhat different to NHL (Ward & Weiss 1989). The progress of Hodgkin's disease is less aggressive, and treatment delay, particularly in the third trimester, may be considered to avoid any fetal risk. In this situation early delivery followed by complete staging and appropriate chemotherapy/radiation therapy should be the management plan. For patients with Hodgkin's disease diagnosed in the first trimester, a delay in commencing treatment until after organogenesis is complete should be considered unless the situation is life-threatening. Thereafter chemotherapy can be used successfully, avoiding agents with a high risk of fetal abnormalities (e.g. procarbazine). In selected cases the use of limited field radiation therapy may be considered to supradiaphragmatic areas.

MISCELLANEOUS TUMOURS

Other less common cancers observed during pregnancy, including cancers of the thyroid, colon, vagina and melanoma, are best managed by surgical treatment as in the non-pregnant patient. In the case of thyroid carcinoma, radioactive iodine and radiation therapy should be deferred until after delivery. Where these cancers are disseminated or metastatic at diagnosis, chemotherapy is of limited effectiveness and if possible the fetus should not be exposed to unnecessary risk.

TRANSPLACENTAL METASTASES

Reports of maternal malignancy involving the placenta and fetus are rare. In a review of the literature Dildy et al (1989) noted that a total of 53 cases had been reported from 1866–1987. Of interest, maternal tumours most likely to be associated with transplacental metastases were not the common tumours seen in pregnancy such as breast or cervical cancer. Among the 53 cases reported malignant melanoma (58%) and leukaemia (33%) accounted for the majority of maternal cancers.

SUMMARY

Cancer during pregnancy is fortunately a rare event. When it occurs both the parents and the physicians are under great stress. Because of its rarity strict management guidelines are difficult to define. The decisions on patient treatment should be a team responsibility involving many different specialities and the parents of the child. In most instances treatment of the cancer and delivery of a healthy child can be achieved. Long-term follow-up of the children should be carried out (Aviles et al 1991; Aviles et al 1988; Sutton et al 1990).

REFERENCES

Allen H, Nisker J 1986 Cancer in pregnancy: An overview. In Allen H, Nisker J (eds) Cancer in Pregnancy – Therapeutic Guidelines. Futura, Mount Kisco, NY, pp 3–7

Aviles A, Niz J 1988 Long-term follow–up of children born to mothers with acute leukemia during pregnancy. Med Pediatr Oncol 16: 3–6

Aviles A, Diaz-Maqueo J C, Talavera A et al 1991 Growth and development of children of mothers treated with chemotherapy during pregnancy: current status of 43 children. Amer J Hemat 36: 243–248

Beeley L 1986 Adverse effects of drugs in the first trimester of pregnancy. Clin Obstet Gynaecol 13: 177–195

Catanzarite V A, Ferguson J E 1984 Acute leukemia and pregnancy: A review of management and outcome, 1972–1982. Obstet Gynecol Surv 39: 663–678

Clark R M, Chua T 1989 Breast cancer and pregnancy: The ultimate challenge. Clin Oncol 1: 11–18

Daly P A, Donnellan P 1992 Breast cancer and pregnancy. Ir Med J 85: 128–130

Dara P, Slater L M, Armentrout S A 1981 Successful pregnancy during chemotherapy for acute leukemia. Cancer 47: 845–846

Dildy III G A, Moise Jr K J, Carpenter Jr R J, Klima T 1989 Maternal malignancy metastatic to the products of conception: a review. Obstet Gynecol Surv 44: 535–539

Doll D C, 1992 Chemotherapy in pregnancy. In Perry M C (ed) The Chemotherapy Source-Book. Williams & Williams, Baltimore, MD, pp 703–709

Doll D C, Ringenberg Q S, Yarbo J W 1988 Management of cancer during pregnancy. Arch Int Med 148: 2058–2064

Doll D C, Ringenberg Q S, Yarbo J W 1989 Antineoplastic agents and pregnancy. Semin Oncol 16: 337–346

Gallenberg M M, Loprinzi C L 1989 Breast cancer and pregnancy. Semin Oncol 16: 369–376

Hopkins M, Morley G W 1992 The prognosis and management of cervical cancer associated with pregnancy. Proc ASCO 11 (Abs): 236

Ioachim H L 1985 Non-Hodgkin's Lymphoma in pregnancy: Three cases and review of the literature. Arch Pathol Lab Med 109: 803–809

Jolles C J 1989 Gynecologic cancer associated with pregnancy. Semin Oncol 16: 417–424

Jones S E, Stringer C A, Dorr R T 1991 Cancer treatment in pregnant women. Educational Book: ASCO 227–238

Nugent P, O'Connell T X 1985 Breast cancer and pregnancy. Arch Surg 120: 1221–1224

Parente J T, Amsel M, Lerner R, Chinea F 1988 Breast cancer associated with pregnancy. Obstet Gynecol 71: 861–864

Petrek J A 1987 Breast cancer and pregnancy. In: Harris J R (ed) Breast Diseases. Lippincott, Philadelphia, pp 600–608

Petrek J A, Dukoff R, Rogatko A 1991 Prognosis of pregnancy-associated breast cancer. Cancer 67: 869–872

Carcinoma of the cervix in pregnancy. 1992 In: Perez C, Brady L (eds) Principles and Practice of Radiation Oncology. Lippincott, Philadelphia, pp 1191–1202

Pizzuto J, Aviles A, Noriega L, et al 1980 Treatment of acute leukemia during pregnancy: Presentation of nine cases. Cancer Treat Rep 64: 679–683

Reynoso E E, Shepherd F A, Messner H A et al 1987 Acute leukemia during pregnancy: The Toronto leukemia group experience with long-term follow-up of children exposed in utero to chemotherapeutic agents. J Clin Oncol 5: 1098–1106

Steiner-Salz D, Yahalom J, Samuelov A, Polliack A 1985 Non-Hodgkin's lymphoma associated with pregnancy: A report of six cases, with a review of the literature. Cancer 8: 2087–2091

Sutcliffe S B, Chapman R M 1986 Lymphomas and leukaemias. In: Allen H H, Nisker J (eds) Cancer in Pregnancy. Futura, Mt. Kisco, NY, pp 135–188

Sutton R, Buzdar A U, Hortobagyi G N 1990 Pregnancy and offspring after adjuvant chemotherapy in breast cancer patients. Cancer 65: 847–850

Theriault R, Walters R, Holmes F et al 1992 Management of breast cancer (BC) during pregnancy (PG). Proc ASCO 11 (Abs): 86

Ward F T, Weiss R B 1989 Lymphoma and pregnancy. Semin Oncol 16: 397–409

Willemse P H B, van der Sijde R, Sleijfer D T H 1990 Combination chemotherapy and radiation for Stage IV breast cancer during pregnancy. Gynecol Oncol 36: 281–284

Zemlickis D, Lishner M, Degendorfer P et al 1992 Maternal and fetal outcome after breast cancer in pregnancy. Am J Obstet Gynecol 166: 781–787

7

Audit in obstetrics

J. Chapple

WHAT IS AUDIT?

Clinical audit is not a new concept – Florence Nightingale drew up 'Forms of Enquiry' in 1828 to look at standards of care in workhouses which later revolutionized nursing – but audit is currently a growth industry. The sum of £41 243 000 was allocated for clinical audit for the National Health Service in the UK in 1993/94. The recent revival of interest in audit arose because professionals, politicians and the public are increasingly concerned with the quality of all public sector services. All are less inclined to accept professional autonomy and paternalism ('Do this because I think it will be good for you') without question. Patients need reassurance that professionals are examining and refining their own practices so that care is constantly and consistently improving. Audit is one method of ensuring that clinicians can rightly take a professional pride in their own work.

The British Government White Paper *Working for Patients* described audit as 'the systematic, critical analysis of the quality of medical care, including the procedures used for diagnosis and treatment, the use of resources and the resulting outcome for the patient' (Secretaries of State 1990). A simpler way of defining audit is to look at it as a set of questions– What do we think we are doing? What are we really doing? How can we improve what we are doing? (Barron 1991) (Table 7.1).

THE AUDIT TEAM

The starting point of any audit is the establishment of a team of workers who have the common purpose of making the audit succeed. The *Oxford English Dictionary* definitions of teams include 'two or more beasts of burden harnessed together' and 'set of players on one side in some games' – which may feel familiar to health service workers. The final definition includes 'combined effort, organized co-operation' – in other words, a group of people coming together to get things done (Firth-Cozens 1992).

Table 7.1 Requirements for clinical audit

- Audit should have the objective to improve the quality of care doctors provide for their patients
- Audit should be systematic and structured
- Audit should use quantitative methods
- Audit should result in change where appropriate, in organization or care provision therefore
- Audit should include follow-up to ensure implementation of results
- Audit should include a record of meetings held, with attendance recorded and a note of subjects covered and recommendations made
- Audit should be undertaken by all doctors and colleges should consider what actions should be directed towards persistent non attenders; however
- Audit should be confidential, educational, and not disciplinary

Standing Medical Advisory Subcommittee, Department of Health 1990 The quality of medical care. London: HMSO

The characteristics of teamwork are:

- Common goals
- Diversity of skills and knowledge
- Support for team members
- Acceptance and management of conflict
- Development of individuals
- Working towards unity.

Belbin (1981) described the different roles played by different personalities in a team. These include:

- A *leader* – to promote discussion, appreciate conflict, and work towards unity.
- *Questioners* – a devil's advocate role to see beyond the detail of the current audit.
- A *link with the outside world* – to ensure the team fits with the needs of larger organizations.
- *Team workers* – to do the jobs between meetings.
- A *finisher* – to concentrate on the end product and get the job done.

A little thought given to forming an audit team may avert possible conflicts and ensure that the key players who can make the process successful are involved.

THE AUDIT CYCLE

No paper on audit would be complete without mention of the audit cycle. Audit requires ownership by the clinical team to think through each stage of the cycle carefully if they want to complete the cycle successfully. The stages of the audit cycle are discussed below (Fig. 7.1).

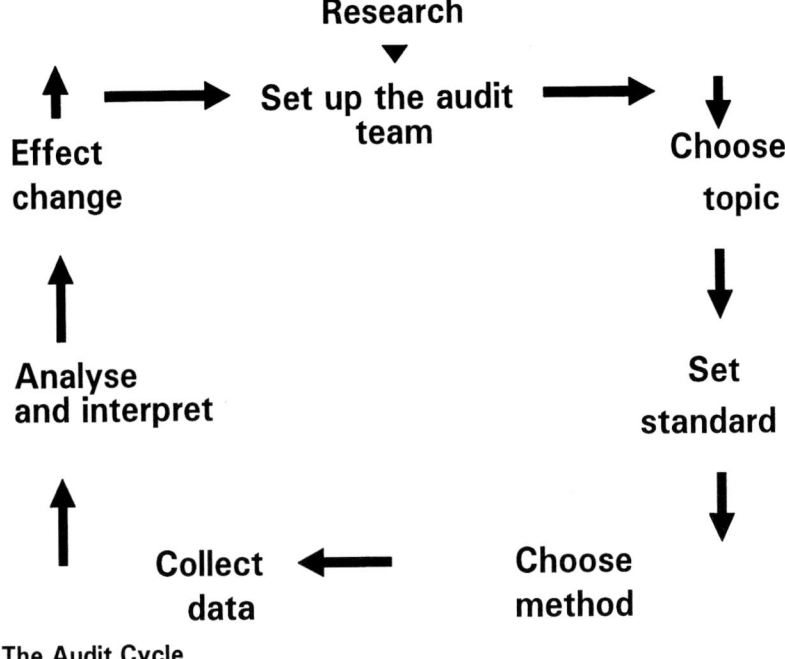

The Audit Cycle

Fig. 7.1 The audit cycle.

Choose a topic

Members of the clinical team need to agree and precisely define a topic for audit – preferably a subject which has aroused debate or concern and is relevant and interesting for the team. This will usually be a topic which occurs commonly – for example, management of early pregnancy loss (Bigrigg & Read 1991), or one which uses a considerable amount of resources, such as infection after Caesarean section (Mugford et al 1989). Successful audit teams should start on the RUMBA (Relevant, Understandable, Measurable, Behaviourly orientated and Achievable) and KISS (Keep It Small and Simple) principles so that they have a good chance of completing the audit.

Maxwell (1984) identified six dimensions of quality, which may be useful in deciding which aspects of a service to audit:

- Access to services
- Relevance to need for the whole community
- Effectiveness for individual clients
- Equity
- Social acceptability
- Efficiency.

Set standards

Standards of clinical care come from two sources: the opinions of health professionals, (normative standards) and the actual practice of such professionals (empirical standards)(Donabedian 1969). It may be extremely difficult to agree on what constitutes a standard of care or management and to set criteria against which performance can be judged. The *Cochrane Collaboration Pregnancy and Childbirth Database* consists of over 600 systematic, regularly updated reviews of randomized trials of care in pregnancy and childbirth. It is available on disc and updated twice yearly. The database can be used to give an idea of the scientific basis (or lack of scientific basis) of clinical practice and to set standards – although good practical decisions rely on more than good reviews of trials.

The audit team needs to agree what levels of compliance with the agreed criteria it is aiming at – does the team want to achieve a minimum level of compliance or try to ensure there is full compliance? Many factors can affect the degree of conformity with criteria and these should be taken into account when setting standards, especially if nationally agreed criteria and protocols are being used. Uncertainty and variability on the outcomes of interventions and about patient's preferences for these outcomes means that standards have to allow some flexibility. There is often a valid rationale for a criterion not being adhered to in particular circumstances.

Choose a method

Donabedian (1966) suggests that there are three areas of clinical care which can be audited:

Structure – the actual facilities provided such as the physical and personnel resources of an organization, including finance.
Process – the way in which these resources are applied. It is concerned with the intervention or treatment and the actions of all those involved– has 'good' practice occurred?
Outcome – the results of health care for the patient.

Ideally an audit of the quality of clinical care should focus on the difference between the outcome desired and that which actually occurs. However, at present there is little research-based evidence to indicate appropriate outcome measures (Shaw 1980) The majority of audits therefore look at the process of care.

Most audit is done retrospectively rather than concurrently, looking back over care given over a set period. This has advantages in that care may temporarily improve if staff know which aspects are being examined closely – but changes to practice because of the Hawthorn effect do not often last.

Using a variety of methods for audit is educational and can enliven the process. Methods include (Maresh 1994):

Basic clinical audit – clinical indicators, routinely collected data

These data are often available from computerized information systems and include perinatal mortality rates (preferably birthweight specific and for normally formed infants), Caesarean section, induction and other intervention rates, length of postoperative stay. These may form the basis of comparative audit, where maternity units compare intervention rates. Those units with values at the limits of the distribution of rates subsequently conduct a more detailed audit to look for the reasons of variation (Paterson et al 1991).

Topic audit – criterion based

This is a relatively labour-intensive method to introduce, so units may want to see if protocols for such audits already exist for local modification. The Medical Audit Unit of the Royal College of Obstetricians and Gynaecologists acts as a clearing house for such protocols. The audit team should pick 10 to 15 questions on the topic to be audited, easily answered by 'yes' or 'no'. For example, a multicentre audit of the management of induced abortion in Scotland used a national consensus survey to agree 15 audit criteria. These included ascertainment of the woman's Rhesus status, maximum waiting times for initial assessment and for operation and availability of choice between a medical or surgical termination for women presenting before 9 weeks gestation (Penney et al 1993, 1994). Once the questions have been formulated, an audit assistant can identify suitable cases and abstract the answers to the questions onto a form for analysis. As with any form of audit, it is essential that confidentiality of both the individual doctors and patients concerned with both 'good' and 'bad' care is preserved.

Random notes, peer review

An independent peer clinician reviews a set of notes picked at random and presents comments. This is a relatively quick and easy method and will give some idea of whether clinical records are kept adequately for retrospective review. However, this type of review may miss major issues and may concentrate on specific rather than general issues – why a particular junior doctor acted inappropriately on a cardiotocograph (CTG) rather than whether appropriate continuing medical education on CTGs is available for all staff.

Critical incident monitoring, adverse patient events, occurrence screening

This is an outcome-based method of audit, looking at adverse outcomes such as perinatal death and return to theatre after operative delivery (Bennett

& Walshe 1990). It mirrors the larger national audits of maternal mortality and the Confidential Enquiry into Stillbirths and Deaths in Infancy (CESDI) in identifying 'avoidable factors' through peer review. If this method is to be successful, it is essential that audit meetings concerning adverse events do not end up as public witch-hunts and that changes in practice aimed at avoiding such adverse outcomes in the future are generally rather than specifically applied.

Collect, analyse and interpret data

Obstetric care is particularly suited to data collection by computer. Pregnancy has a definite start and finish and a defined outcome – the birth of a child. There is also a limited number of complications or comorbidities which affect pregnancy. It is therefore easy to collect routine data on each pregnancy, whether by coding or capture of raw data as the woman proceeds through the various stages of maternity care. Computers are a particularly good way to organize data collection, ensuring that information on large numbers of cases can be accessed easily and quickly in the maternity unit itself. Several computer packages for collecting and organizing data already exist – the St Mary's Maternity Information System (Paterson et al 1991) and Euro King systems, for example. All units should have access to some baseline statistics on the maternity care they provide from the maternity Hospital Episode Systems (HES) data set.

A good database does make it possible to identify particular groups of cases for detailed study and, with a few additional items, can be used for audit (Yudkin & Redman 1990). However, lack of a computer or computer literacy should not be a deterrent to audit. Judicious use of pen and paper makes it possible to audit all aspects of maternity services without a computer package, using data collected in notebooks and registers. It is important to analyse and interpret data obtained from handwritten records frequently and in small amounts, or a large mound of information will collect that no one will relish sorting and analysing.

It must be remembered that any method of collecting and analysing data provides a means of identifying the need for change, and is not the purpose of the audit in itself. The final part of the audit cycle is the most important, and potentially the most difficult.

Effect change

People, including clinicians, do not behave in an entirely rational, scientific way and do not automatically change practice when given good evidence that there may be a more effective way of providing care (Stocking 1992). However, clinicians want to do what is best for their patients, but often disagree about what 'the best' actually is – as Ogden Nash puts it, 'I believe that people believe what they believe they believe'. There are sins of omission – things that should be done which are not – and sins of commission – things that are done that should not be done.

There are five characteristics of innovation which affect the adoption of a different practice, each of which may be considered differently by each individual who needs to be involved in producing change (Rogers 1983):

- It is not only the outcome for the patient that influences whether one practice is perceived as having a **relative advantage** over another – for example, it may need new skills, increase or decrease income or reassure professionals. What is seen as advantageous by one group may be perceived as disadvantageous to others. For example, routine induction of labour was seen as beneficial to professionals and to some women, but not accepted by others.
- Some changes may be incompatible with current beliefs, philosophy or working practices. Changes in the general environment may be needed to produce **compatibility** before more specific changes can be achieved.
- If change needs involvement of disparate groups, then the **complexity** of negotiations will affect the ability to change as each individual's prestige and influence may be affected. However, this sort of change tends to stick – so many people have been involved and have needed to compromise and adapt their philosophies that there is no going back. Conversely, changes which are relatively simple may be adopted quickly, but there may be a gradual reversion to old practices if the 'change champion' leaves.
- **Observability** (can you see change?) and **trialability** (can you try it out on a limited basis?) are the last two characteristics of innovation which may be considered when formulating plans to complete the audit cycle. Both tend to encourage changes in practice as they allow some flexibility.

Strategies which have been tried in promoting change in clinical practice include:

Education – vocational and continuing.   Audit and education are inextricably linked – undergraduates need to learn about audit in order to appreciate that medicine is not a pure science and that there are no 'right' answers to anything. Staff can be educated by audit and it may well identify educational needs – for example, training in the interpretation of CTG scans, with acknowledgement that if a CTG appears abnormal, something more needs to be done than to change the CTG machine and leave it in the corridor for someone else to use.

Peer review and patient pressure.   This should theoretically lead to person-to-person contact with respected peers or opinion leaders and alter practice through peer pressure. Lomas et al (1991) found that most studies achieving change through audit were concerned with laboratory testing, diagnostic radiology, and drug prescribing rather than medical or surgical practice. This study used two strategies to try to increase the use of trial of labour and vaginal delivery after a single previous Caesarean section – audit and feedback of information (which achieved no change in practice) and intervention by local medical opinion leaders to encourage colleagues to change practice by talking to them and organizing educational activities (which increased vaginal delivery rates).

Well informed patients can also influence practice – an example from Switzerland showed that a media campaign in appropriate languages in one canton lowered the rates of hysterectomy compared with those in other cantons where a campaign had not been mounted (Domenighetti et al 1988).

Financial incentives are a means of producing change, as the achievement of target rates for cervical cytology after payment to general practitioners shows. A cynic may add that change induced by money may be irrespective of whether there is good evidence of improvement of clinical outcome, and actually discourages questioning practice. In both Australia and the UK, the intervention rates for Caesarean section and instrumental delivery for private patients are nearly double those for women giving birth in public hospitals, with no evidence to show that these higher intervention rates confer any improvement in outcome for the mother or her baby (King 1993).

Passively providing information about the results of research and feedback on individual practice is unlikely to produce change unless it is linked to audit and educational processes (Mugford et al 1991). It is therefore important that feedback is active, so attention needs to be given to making the ubiquitous audit meeting effective.

AUDIT MEETINGS

It is essential that all concerned have an opportunity to comment on the audit findings – clinicians will be more willing to change if they feel they have ownership of the data. This is usually done through audit meetings.

Jay (1976) reviews ways of running business meetings to make them effective, which reverberate for successful audit meetings where change must be planned. The paper suggests that the chairman for a productive meeting must actively control the proceedings and will:

• Control the garrulous
• Draw out the silent
• Protect the weak
• Encourage the clash of ideas
• Watch out for the suggestion-squashing reflex
• Come to the most senior people last
• Close on a note of achievement.

It is vital that meetings have a chairman who chairs, use clinicians other than doctors to present data when the audit is multidisciplinary and that proposed changes are written down and disseminated widely, preferably in the form of practice guidelines and protocols. It is also vital to repeat the audit at a later date to audit the audit process and see if change has been effected. This is particularly important for hospitals that produce annual reports and hold large report meetings, as the meeting may become an end in itself, focusing on a different topic each year rather than ensuring that practice is changed appropriately.

WHAT AUDIT IS NOT

Reflection on the audit process should clarify the common misconceptions between audit and research. The aim of clinical research is to look for new knowledge of medical care in order to draw conclusions which may be valid in similar clinical circumstances. Research focuses on generating or testing hypotheses and measures the efficacy of treatment. In contrast, the aim of clinical audit is to review clinical care against agreed professional standards in order to identify opportunities for improvement. Clinical audit measures effectiveness of treatment and improves quality and efficiency of clinical care. Research discovers new knowledge or 'the right thing to do' whereas audit seeks to ensure that current knowledge is fully and properly used – 'making sure it is done right' (Table 7.2).

ISSUES ABOUT AUDIT IN OBSTETRICS

Obstetrics is a rare clinical specialty in that it deals in the main with a normal and natural physiological process rather than an illness. For this reason, audit in obstetrics differs from many other types of audit as discussed below.

Table 7.2   How research differs from audit

Research
- May involve experiments on human subjects, whether patients, patients as volunteers or health volunteers
- Is a systematic investigation which aims to increase the sum of knowledge
- May involve allocating patients randomly to different treatment groups
- May involve a completely new treatment
- May involve extra disturbance or work beyond that required for normal clinical management
- Usually involves an attempt to test an hypothesis
- May involve the application of strict selection criteria to patients with the same problem before they are entered into the research study

Audit
- Never involves experiments, whether on healthy volunteers or patients as volunteers
- Is a systematic approach to the peer review of clinical care in order to identify opportunities for improvement and to provide a mechanism for bringing them about
- Never involves allocating patients randomly to different treatment groups
- Never involves a placebo treatment
- Never involves a completely new treatment
- Never involves disturbance to the patients beyond that required for normal clinical management
- May involve patients with the same problem being given different treatment, but only after full discussion of the known advantages and disadvantages of each treatment. The patients are allowed to choose freely which treatment they get.

Obstetric audit is clinical rather than medical

The majority of pregnancies are looked after by midwives rather than doctors, and a midwife is the senior member of staff present at over 70% of deliveries. It is therefore impossible to conduct any aspect of obstetric audit without the input of this important group of clinicians. Some midwives still work either in acute units or in the community; both groups must be included in the audit. Senior and junior obstetricians must be prepared to involve midwives as equal partners in the audit process, accepting suggestions and constructive criticism from them as well as from other medical staff.

Obstetric audit is multidisciplinary

Many specialties other than obstetrics and midwifery may be involved in routine maternity care. Other specialists who should be involved in at least some aspects of obstetric audit include:

• Gynaecology nurses
• Ultrasonographers and radiologists
• Physiotherapists
• Paediatricians and neonatologists
• Anaesthetists
• Pathologists and pathology technicians
• Geneticists and genetic counsellors
• General practitioners.

It is also important to remember the receptionist if patient views on care are to be included, especially in out-patients. If patients are involved, confidentiality must be ensured to obtain the real views of women, which are unlikely to be given if the completed questionnaire is handed directly to the receptionist – either use a collection box by the door or distribute stamped addressed envelopes. It goes without saying that any patient questionnaires must use easy-to-understand language, with special thought given as to how to gather the views of non-English speaking patients.

Much maternity care takes place in the community prior to delivery

Obstetric audit should cover:

• Primary care and community services: pre-pregnancy advice, antenatal care, home or GP unit deliveries and postnatal care outside hospital.
• Secondary care: antenatal care, antenatal diagnosis, delivery and postnatal care, routine neonatal care in hospital.
• Tertiary care: referrals to specialist centres for antenatal diagnosis, care of problems such as severe hypertension at early gestations, neonatal intensive or surgical care and intra- or extra-uterine transfers for such care.

Pregnant women are informed consumers of care

The consumer revolution which has swept through health care in the last decade started in the maternity services. Women often prepare birth plans and are increasingly and rightly involved in decisions about the management of their pregnancy. Good audit projects will pay attention to consumer involvement and satisfaction.

The majority of obstetricians also see gynaecology patients

They therefore need to audit their work in this field as well as their obstetric work. Very few other clinicians have two such large and differing groups of patients. Time available for audit in obstetrics by doctors is therefore likely to be strictly rationed. Involvement of midwives and audit facilitators and assistants may help with this problem.

SOURCES OF INFORMATION FOR OBSTETRIC AUDIT

Cochrane pregnancy and childbirth database

The National Perinatal Epidemiology Unit started to compile a register of references to randomized controlled trials in 1978. The register stemmed from the belief that data which are already available should be fully exploited before resources are committed to the collection of additional information. The register is now available on computer disc and comprises references to over 600 published reports of randomized controlled trials and details of many other unpublished, ongoing and planned trials in the field of perinatal medicine. The database has been used to produce overviews (meta analyses) of the results of randomized controlled trials – in other words, similar trials are incorporated in a single analysis to draw statistically valid conclusions on the effectiveness of interventions such as corticosteroids given to women expected to deliver preterm, vacuum extraction versus forceps delivery, etc. This can be a useful guide to setting scientific standards for maternity care. The computer database is available from:

BMJ Publishing Group
PO Box 295
London WC1H 9TE
Tel (+44) 0171 383 6185/6245
Fax (+44) 0171 383 6662

The first comprehensive collection of these systematic reviews was published in 1989 in a 1500 page, two volume hardback book called *Effective care in pregnancy and childbirth* (commonly known as ECPC) (Chalmers et al 1989) and in an inexpensive paperback edition – *A guide to effective care in pregnancy and childbirth* (Chalmers et al 1994).

Obtaining women's views of maternity care

The Department of Health commissioned a very detailed questionnaire and analysis package from the Office of Population Censuses and Surveys (OPCS) which examines women's views on all aspects of their maternity care. The questionnaire has been fully validated and can be used in its entirety or to cover selected areas of care. Both *Womens' experience of maternity care* and *Getting the consumer's view of maternity care* can be obtained from Her Majesty's Stationery Office (HMSO) 24 hour telephone ordering service (+44) 0171 873 9090.

Partograms

The majority of hospital obstetric units use partograms to summarize all the events occurring in labour. Where these have been accurately and completely kept they provide an easy source of information on intrapartum events for collection by nonclinical staff such as audit assistants.

Routine statistics

As mentioned above, all units should be able to obtain information on total deliveries, operative deliveries, etc. from the maternity Hospital Episode System (HES) data set. Data on pregnancies are also readily available from national data collection systems:

Birth notification.   All deliveries must be notified by one of the birth attendants (usually a midwife) to the local Director of Public Health within 36 hours of the birth. This includes the gestational age at delivery, birthweight, and any congenital malformations diagnosed at birth. Notification is often used to start off the *child health record* on a child health computer system. There is therefore the potential to link obstetric data with longer-term outcomes in childhood.

Notification data are passed to the local registrar of births and deaths for inclusion in the *birth registration* system, which records demographic details from parents. Birth registration data are collated to provide information by geographical area of residence of the mother by OPCS. Routine statistics, like all others, are only as good as the figures fed into them via clinical staff. A good starting point for local audit might be to check the completeness and accuracy of notification data (such as information on congenital malformations) and improve reporting if deficits are found.

KEY AUDITS IN OBSTETRICS

National confidential enquiry into maternal deaths

Reports from this voluntary but complete form of adverse event audit have been published every 3 years by HMSO since 1952 and provide guidelines on issues which still cause deaths in mothers. There was concern that the enquiry was not producing change as it relied on passive feedback of pooled anonymous data, and recently there have been efforts to ensure that recommendations in the reports are acted on and protocols for dealing with potentially fatal complications are available (Patel 1992).

National confidential enquiry into stillbirths and deaths in infancy (CESDI)

A few regional surveys and confidential enquiries into perinatal deaths have been running since the late 1970s. All English Regions were required to set up stillbirth and infant death surveys from January 1993 under a new Department of Health initiative to set up nationwide adverse event audits – the National Confidential Enquiry into Stillbirths and Deaths in Infancy (CESDI). This includes late fetal deaths from 20 weeks gestation as well as deaths in the first year of life. Different subgroups are targeted for a more detailed investigation by peer review panels. The initial two subgroups for confidential enquiry were intrapartum deaths of normally formed babies of birthweight greater than 2500 g and unexpected deaths in infancy.

Some confidential enquiries include an interview with the mother and/ or father of the dead child to discover the parents' view of what went wrong in the pregnancy. This has been instrumental in improving the quality of bereavement counselling for this group.

Regional congenital malformation registers

Several English health regions now run congenital malformation registers which include abnormal ultrasound reporting and which can be used to audit antenatal screening programmes. There are also national registers for monitoring the incidence of some specific conditions, such as the national Down's syndrome register, based at the Department of Clinical Epidemiology at the London Hospital Medical College (Mutton et al 1991).

National eclampsia survey

For the first time in 1992, all cases of eclampsia occurring in the UK were reported to the British Eclampsia Survey Team (BEST) in Oxford (Douglas & Redman 1994). Eclampsia is still an important cause of maternal and perinatal mortality and morbidity. This study showed that eclampsia complicates nearly 1 in 2000 pregnancies in the UK, with nearly 1 in 50 women dying of the condition, as do 1 in 14 of their babies, despite most eclamptic convulsions occurring in hospital in women who have received antenatal care. It is therefore important that every maternity unit has well-established protocols to avoid delays in the diagnosis and management of eclampsia.

Clinical indicators

Organizations in the United States (the American College of Obstetrics and Gynaecology and the Joint Commission for the Accreditation of Health Care Organizations) have produced lists of clinical indicators for use in obstetrics and neonatology. While the criteria used by these groups may not be wholly suitable for use in the UK, they do provide possible starting points and can be fairly easily adapted in line with accepted British practice. Work has also been done in Australia to produce criteria for clinical care.

LITIGATION AND AUDIT

Obstetrics is a highly litigious specialty and in the past many cases have proved difficult to defend as a result of poor quality of the records, or to genuine faults in practice which may be partly caused by poor education or supervision or inadequate guidelines. Most hospitals are setting up risk management schemes for all specialties. Obstetrics plays a key role because of the considerable amounts awarded to successful plaintiffs. Audit of litigation is important, but adverse event reporting is only a small part of good obstetric audit. Effective audit of all aspects of care should improve the quality of clinical records and the level of education of all staff. The results may be used to draw up clear guidelines for management of difficult areas. This in turn should help to protect against litigation in the future.

WILL AUDIT WORK?

Mugford & Chapple (1993) reviewed the effect of recent changes in the National Health Service on perinatal audit and concluded that:

- The culture within units will determine the priority given to audit – but this may be helped by adequate backup from audit staff and well supported routine information systems.
- Purchasers will need to specify the need for audit results in their contracts with providers so that there is a possibility of the loss of contracts if good audit activity does not occur.
- Unless good quality statistical information is easily available, audit cannot advance from the isolated one-off studies to which it is usually confined at present.

SOURCES OF HELP FOR AUDIT

The Royal College of Obstetricians and Gynaecologists (RCOG) Audit Unit has established a database of successful audit protocols and have themselves devised protocols for audit of a number of areas in obstetrics, including Caesarean sections, instrumental deliveries and the management of term babies who required special care. They have also utilized the information available in the Cochrane Pregnancy and Childbirth database to produce a list of procedures known to be effective which can be used to draw up standards for audit. A package containing the protocols, list of effective procedures, American and Australian audit criteria and other useful information, as well as help with all areas of audit (including the analysis of results from Audit Unit protocols) is available from:

RCOG Audit Unit
St Mary's Hospital
Hathersage Road
Whitworth Park
Manchester M13 OJH
Telephone (+44) 0161 276 6300, fax (+44) 0161 276 6311.

KEY POINTS FOR SUCCESSFUL CLINICAL AUDIT

1. Audit needs a defined condition to be studied, an agreed standard of practice, established measures of process or outcome and easy access to data for collection. It also needs a critical mass of clinicians and resources, usually enthusiasm, time, people and money.

2. Resources for audit are earned by specifying good projects. Find the local infrastructure (such as a helpful audit assistant) to support you in an audit project.

3. Audit your own practice and choose as a topic something you can change. If it is likely that a change in practice is needed from others, involve them from the start.

4. Start small so you get somewhere quickly. You need early achievement to maintain interest.

5. Choose a topic on an agreed area of importance e.g. high mortality, risk, cost or one where there is total disagreement. National audits, such as confidential enquiries can act as bench marks for local audit.

6. Differentiate audit from research – audit is about the application of already established best practice.

7. Make sure the audit cycle is completed, that change in practice has occurred and has the effects predicted.

8. Obstetric audit is multidisciplinary and must involve professionals other than doctors and also consumers of care.

9. Link audit with continuing education for all professionals.

10. Some things cannot be answered by audit.

REFERENCES

Barron S L 1991 Audit in obstetrics. Br J Obstet Gynaecol 98: 1065–1072
Belbin R M 1981 Management realms: why they succeed or fail. Halstead Press, New York
Bennett J, Walshe K 1990 Occurrence screening as a method of audit. Br Med J 300: 1248–1251
Bigrigg M A, Read M D 1991 Management of women referred to early pregnancy assessment unit: care and cost effectiveness. Br Med J 302: 577–579
Chalmers I, Enkin M, Keirse M J N C 1989 Effective care in pregnancy and childbirth. Oxford University Press, Oxford
Chalmers I, Enkin M, Keirse M J N C 1994 A guide to effective care in pregnancy and childbirth. 2nd edition. Oxford University Press, Oxford
Domenighetti G, Luraschi P, Casabianca A et al 1988 Effect of information campaign by the mass media on hysterectomy rates. Lancet ii: 1470–1473
Donabedian A 1966 Evaluating the quality of medical care. Milbank Mem Fund Q Part 2 44: 166–206
Donabedian A 1969 A guide to medical care administration. Volume II: Medical care appraisal – quality and utilization. The American Public Health Association, Washington.
Douglas K A, Redman C W G 1994 Eclampsia in the United Kingdom. Br Med J 309: 1395–1400
Firth-Cozens J 1992 Building teams for effective audit. Quality in Health Care 1: 252–255
Jay A 1976 How to run a meeting. Harvard Business Review 54: 43–57
King J F 1993 Obstetric intervention and the economic imperative. Br J Obstet Gynaecol 100: 303–306
Lomas J, Enkin M, Anderson G M et al 1991 Opinion leaders vs audit and feedback to implement practice guidelines. JAMA 265: 2202–2207
Maresh M 1994 Audit in obstetrics and gynaecology. Blackwell Scientific Publications, Oxford
Maxwell R J 1984 Quality assessment in health. Br Med J 288: 1470–1473
Mugford M, Chapple J 1993 How have recent changes in the NHS affected perinatal audit? Arch Dis Child 69: 322–326
Mugford M, Kingston J, Chalmers I 1989 Reducing the incidence of infection after Caesarean section: implications of prophylaxis with antibiotics for hospital resources. Br Med J 299: 1003–1006
Mugford M, Banfield P, O'Hanlon M 1991 The effects of feedback of information on clinical practice: a review. Br Med J 303: 398–402
Mutton D E, Alberman E, Ide R et al 1991 Results of the first year (1989) of a national register of Down's syndrome in England and Wales. Br Med J 303: 1295–1297
OPCS 1989 Womens' experience of maternity care. Her Majesty's Stationery Office, London
OPCS 1993 Getting the consumer's view of maternity care. Her Majesty's Stationery Office, London
Patel N 1992 Maternal mortality – the way forward. Royal College of Obstetries and Gynaecology, London
Paterson C M, Chapple J C, Beard R W et al 1991 Evaluating the quality of the maternity services – a discussion paper. Br J Obstet Gynaecol 98: 1073–1078
Penney G C, Glasier A, Templeton A 1993 Agreeing criteria for audit of management of induced abortion: an approach by national consensus survey. Quality in Health Care 2: 167–169
Penney G C, Glasier A, Templeton A 1994 Multicentre criterion based audit of the management of induced abortion in Scotland. Br Med J 309: 15–19
Rogers B 1983 Attributes of innovation and their rate of adaptation. In: Rogers B (ed) Diffusion of innovations. 3rd edition. Free Press, New York pp. 210–240
Secretaries of State for Health, Wales, Northern Ireland and Scotland. 1990 Working for patients. Working paper number 6. 'Medical audit'. Her Majesty's Stationery Office, London

Shaw C D 1980 Aspects of audit: I. The background. Br Med J 280: 1256–1258
Standing Medical Advisory Subcommittee, Department of Health 1990 The quality of medical care. Her Majesty's Stationery Office, London
Stocking B 1992 Promoting change in clinical care. Quality in Health Care 1: 56–60
Yudkin P L, Redman C W G 1990 Obstetric audit using routinely collected computerized data. Br Med J 301: 1371–1373

8

Avoiding complications in minimally invasive pelvic surgery

S. Duffy

This chapter should not be read as a prescriptive list of do's and don'ts of endoscopic surgery, but as a basis for discussion and a way to heighten awareness of the complexities of what is becoming an ever-expanding area of gynaecological practice. Bearing in mind the restrictions on space and the large subject content to cover, in-depth discussion, by necessity, is impossible. A working knowledge of the techniques of hysteroscopy and laparoscopy are therefore assumed. The format of the chapter is that of brief practicality.

It is interesting to follow the historical development of endoscopy in gynaecology and see how the enquiring minds of gynaecologists have, to a greater or lesser extent, led the developments in this field. Undoubtedly, improvements in equipment design have been part of the development process, the relationship between industry and medical practice being symbiotic in nature. As the technology is stretched, so too are the limits of clinical application. At each stage, as the boundaries are pushed forward, there has been, and always will be, a component of danger. It behoves all who operate in any surgical speciality to learn how far to push and to set one's own limitations.

Hysteroscopy started life as a means of observing the uterine cavity. With poor light and no distension in the earlier stages, it is remarkable that the technique was not abandoned. As rod lens systems (Hopkins 1953) and better light sources became available, hysteroscopy came of age. By using distension to aid visualization proper diagnosis became possible. Refinements in distension were to follow, a classic example of which was setting the safety limits of CO_2 distension. Fluid media for distension, especially the latest continuous-flow system, have come close to the optimum requirement for complete and safe visualization of the interior of the uterine cavity. These changes have resulted from the need to prevent complications. Once the limitations of visualization were overcome, the path was clear for the development of the therapeutic role of hysteroscopy. With this came a new source of complications – surgery.

Laparoscopy began in the early 1900s, and was initially favoured by physicians. The technique was quickly taken up by gynaecologists and surgeons. The ability to visualize the entire abdominal cavity led to the obvious exploration of therapeutic roles. Tubal sterilization was one of the first procedures described (Bosch 1936), along with the identification of ectopic pregnancy (Hope 1937). Problems with electrosurgery within an oxygen-distended cavity led to the introduction of CO_2 distension, another example of complication leading to improvement in safety. Nowadays, with the increase in surgical expertise, new areas of laparoscopic treatment are being opened up. There is a wealth of new instruments available as manufacturers try to keep pace with the needs of surgeons, and with each new instrument comes the potential for unwanted damage.

Laparoscopy and hysteroscopy literally place the surgeon at arms length from the site of surgery. There is a loss of tactile discrimination and reliance on a two-dimensional perspective. This requires retraining in skills of dexterity and depth perception. The principles of surgical technique, learned in more conventional open surgical practice, are as important in the enclosed confines of the minimally invasive operative field as in the open abdomen. Knowledge of anatomy, relationships of organs, nerve and blood supply become more important when operating in confined spaces. Ancillary technologies, such as laser and electrosurgery, if utilized, must be clearly understood to ensure their safe application.

As a generalization, complications in minimally invasive surgery can be categorized into those relating to: anaesthesia, instrumentation, operator error, and ancillary equipment.

ANAESTHESIA

There is no reason why the majority of patients cannot be offered hysteroscopic assessment, for diagnostic purposes, as ambulant outpatients. This avoids the complications of general anaesthesia. Operative hysteroscopy can also be performed under a mixture of local and sedative anaesthesia (Magos et al 1989) or local anaesthesia alone (Rankin & Steinberg 1992).

If local anaesthesia is used, the surgeon must be aware of the total allowable dose of active compound used (dependent on the concentration of anaesthetic), and also the risk of anaphylaxis. A fully equipped resuscitation trolley should be readily available where patients are being treated. The common site of injection for hysteroscopic cases is para- or intracervical blockade, which facilitates cervical dilatation. Vagal reaction, as a result of cervical dilatation, often requires treatment with intravenous atropine to correct the associated bradycardia.

During laparoscopy, the majority of patients will be operated on under general anaesthesia. The obvious risks relate to the induction and maintenance of patients during the procedure. The anaesthetist is well placed to ensure patient safety during the administration of the anaesthetic. The surgeon must ensure, however, that the anaesthetized patient is placed safely and appropriately on the operating table, avoiding unwanted positional joint or nerve damage. This is especially important with prolonged operative procedures. A further consideration is the distension of the abdominal cavity during laparoscopy. With the relatively high flow rate and large volume of CO_2 used (compared to hysteroscopy) there is a greater risk of CO_2 embolisation. Some anaesthetists will routinely auscultate over the praecordium to detect the machinery murmur associated with this complication.

INSTRUMENTATION

Correct maintenance of telescopes, cameras and light cables will ensure optimum visualization during all endoscopic procedures. Backup equipment is not a luxury but essential in the event of accidental damage.

Distension

Before commencing any endoscopic procedure, equipment checks will prevent the frustration of failure and encourage safe practice. Hysteroscopic CO_2 insufflators, either automatic or manual, have built-in safety features. The integrity of these systems should be checked on every occasion. The flow rate and safety cut-out can be assessed by blocking the outflow tubing. The flow rate should decrease as the pressure gauge level increases. The maximum pressure allowable is up to 200 mm Hg, the maximum flow rate should be 100 ml per minute (Lindemann 1972). Similar pressure and flow alterations are used in fluid-distending systems. During laparoscopic insufflation the same checks should be performed. However, there are additional features relating to laparoscopic gas flow rates and pressures. The flow rate usually starts at 1 L/minute (10 times the rate of hysteroscopic insufflation). This rate should only be increased when the pneumoperitoneum is complete and a cannula has been introduced so that visual confirmation of abdominal entry is confirmed. The rate can then be increased to 4 or 5 L/minute. A guide to intra-abdominal pressure is also provided on most insufflators and the usual maximum setting is at 15 mm Hg. The insufflation pressure is usually between 5–10 mm Hg. This prevents overdistension of the abdominal cavity and inferior vena caval compression.

Low-viscosity fluid distension (such as glycine 1.5%) during continuous-flow hysteroscopy can employ a simple gravity-fed system, where the height of the inflow irrigation solution above the operative site determines the pressure achieved. The outflow often has a small degree of negative pressure attached to it. The mechanical, or pump equivalent to this simple gravity system has an in-built ability of continuous inflow/outflow volume deficit calculation. In addition there are systems available where the intrauterine pressure is titrated against the volume and flow rate instilled (Garry et al 1992). The overriding principle is the prevention of excessive fluid absorption. Prevention and early detection of fluid intravasation during hysteroscopic surgery reduces the risk of fluid overload in the patient. Whichever system is employed there should be one person responsible for the monitoring of instilled fluid in order to warn the operator of approaching fluid overload. At present, a working rule of thumb is that surgery should be stopped if the fluid deficit reaches 2–2.5 L. The rate at which the deficit develops is as important as the absolute value.

High-viscosity fluids (dextran) are associated with anaphylaxis when absorbed. Large volumes of dextran also act as an anticoagulant. If allowed to remain on instruments and not cleaned thoroughly, the dextran can cause the instruments to become permanently sealed.

Hysteroscopy: telescopes and sheaths

Flexible hysteroscopes require careful maintenance as the insufflation channels are narrow and blockage with debris will cause failure in distension and frustration. Fluid disinfection, such as Cidex™, is usually needed for these instruments. Careful rinsing and drying is required to ensure that no residual solution remains prior to use. The patient may develop a dermatitis-type reaction to the local instillation of such material in or adjacent to the cervix or uterus. If sterilizing solution is left in-situ it may also cause bubble formation once gas distension is started and therefore cause obstruction of the surgeon's view. Rigid telescopes are now autoclavable which obviates the need for fluid disinfection.

The outer operating hysteroscopy sheaths all use a system of stopcocks to allow inflow of gas or fluid. These are potential leakage sites which will lead to lack of distension. Also, special sheaths are used for continuous-flow systems with separate inflow and outflow channels. It is essential that the correct inflow and outflow ports are used. Connecting an inflow tube to an outflow sheath will result in inadequate distension and the inability to operate safely. Finally, hysteroresection inner sheaths also have a ceramic beak which acts as an insulator. If this breaks down, either by accident or as a result of continued contact to an activated resection loop, there will be a breach in insulation. This will result in the passage of electrosurgical current to the external sheath of the resectoscope and will be transmitted to the patient and surgeon inadvertently.

Laparoscopy: telescopes, cannulae, veress' needle

The veress' needle relies on the integrity of the spring mechanism to prevent sharp perforation of underlying organs. The mechanism should be checked prior to insertion of the needle. Some disposable needles have a green/red indicator to help identify successful and safe entry. The veress' needle should be checked for patency by connecting the insufflation tubing before use. Blockage may be caused by debris or a kink in the metal shaft.

Laparoscopic cannulae also use stopcocks to enable insufflation. The stopcocks and the rubber seal are potential leakage sites that are easily checked. Newer disposable cannulae are less prone to leakage at these points. If the latter are chosen in preference to the reusable versions, the operator must become familiar with the safety features and operation of the protective sleeve that act in a similar fashion to the veress' needle.

Laparoscopic telescopes often become misty or frosted when first passed through the main portal/cannula. This may obscure the view and can be prevented by prewarming the telescope or by using a secondary port for the insufflating gas (the CO_2 acts as a coolant as it passes through the main cannula, adding to the mist effect).

ANCILLARY INSTRUMENTS

Conventional accessories

Scissors, biopsy and grasping forceps can be disposable or reusable. The advantage of disposable instruments is that there is less likelihood of the instrument being blunt or damaged. Reusable instruments require careful handling to ensure lasting use. The sites of deteriorating function are the sharpness of scissors and the working joints of the graspers. Less than satisfactory instruments will result in tissue tearing and unnecessary trauma with bleeding.

During hysteroscopy, a clear view is maintained by the continuous flow of fluid. The same applies to laparoscopy and the system used is a combined suction/irrigation instrument. In order to clear blood or visualize a bleeding area to control the haemorrhage, a good system of flushing and suction is necessary. The suction is also useful in clearing the smoke plume associated with the use of electrosurgery and laser.

Electrosurgery

There are three considerations if electrosurgery is used during operative endoscopy: the operator, the patient, and the instruments used. The operator must understand the principles of electrosurgery and the relationship between the instruments used, the electrosurgical unit, and the patient (Duffy & Cobb 1994). During electrosurgery the patient forms part of the electrical current circuit. With monopolar electrosurgery the current flows from an active electrode (for example a loop) to a return plate (usually placed on the patient's thigh). With bipolar electrosurgery the current flows from the active tip of a forceps to the passive tip which is immediately adjacent. With monopolar electrosurgery the distance the current travels through the patient is greater than that of bipolar electrosurgery, therefore there is more potential for accidental damage caused by stray current. There is increasing interest in the development of both cutting and coagulating bipolar electrosugery. However, at the moment, monopolar electrosurgery is the most commonly employed modality. The electrosurgical unit that is chosen should comply with national and international safety standards.

Electrosurgery uses the localization of current to achieve the desired effect, either cutting or coagulation. Different current waveforms are used to deliver the current to the tissues.Cutting is achieved with a continuous waveform. Soft or desiccation coagulation is achieved using an intermittent low-peak voltage waveform. Forced or spray coagulation uses an intermittent high-peak voltage waveform. The duration of exposure to the current contributes to the amount of tissue destruction and the production and transmission of thermal energy (Duffy et al 1991, 1992a). Controlling the immediate tissue destruction and the transmission of heat is the responsibility of the operator.

During operative hysteroscopy, monopolar electrosurgery is used for: endometrial ablation with the rollerball, endometrial resection with the loop, or when using a combination of both. Intrauterine septae may be divided with an electrosurgical needle, but adhesions should be removed using conventional instruments such as scissors and forceps. Electrosurgery is an efficient means of destroying tissue and must be guided by the surgeon. For a given tissue the coagulation effect of the rollerball is achieved quickly. The principal factor leading to excessive tissue destruction, especially with the forced or spray coagulation, is time. Therefore prolonged exposure should be avoided. Cutting with a resection loop will have a degree of tissue destruction underlying the loop but the amount of tissue removed will depend on the depth the surgeon takes the loop into the myometrium, therefore caution and knowledge of the allowable depth is essential.

Laparoscopy provides ample opportunity for inadvertent damage using electrosurgery. Monopolar electrosurgery is the commonest modality used for cutting and coagulating, but increasingly bipolar devices are appearing. The benefit of bipolar electrosurgery is the short distance between the electrodes, thus allowing visual control over the electrosurgical effect. Also the tissue between the electrodes is the only part of the patient involved in the circuit, thereby minimizing the potential for unwanted damage. Electrosurgical current will always pass along the path of least resistance from its active to its passive electrode. This includes passage along a thin adhesion, for example, with possible transmission to bowel if attached to one end of the adhesion. As a guide, any area being treated by electrosurgery should be held clear of any other tissue if possible. The area should be viewed as a panorama rather than close up so that all adjoining structures are in the field of view. The active electrode and treated area are momentarily hot after application of the electrode and should be cautiously replaced to avoid contact with the bowel.

There are three main hazards with electrosurgical instruments: direct electrical coupling, insulation breakdown, and capacitance coupling.

Direct coupling is inadvertent contact of an active electrode with tissue. During laparoscopy more than one instrument may be in the abdominal cavity at any one time. With two or more long instruments in place there is a risk of each of the instruments touching each other. If an active electrode touches a telescope, the telescope will conduct the current and transmit it to any tissue in contact, for example the bowel. Insulation breakdown in any electrosurgical forceps is very serious as the failure usually occurs out of view of the operator. A leak of current at any point along a forceps will potentially lead to tissue damage in adjacent structures. Capacitance coupling occurs where two electrical conductors are separated by an insulating layer, for example an active electrode surrounded by its insulated layer and placed in a metal cannula. The build-up of current will, in this example, occur on the surface of the cannula. If sufficient, the current build up can be discharged to nearby tissue and cause a burn. Recent advances in the technology have reduced the risk of these complications. An electrical current detector (Electroshield™) fits over the electrosurgical electrode and will sense any alterations of current flow as a result of insulation breakdown or capacitance (Odell 1993). The instrument can then alarm and shut down the electrosurgical unit to prevent damage.

A recent innovation in electrosurgical equipment is the argon-beam coagulator. This instrument provides a high-flow stream of argon gas to the operation site. Piggy-backed onto this stream of gas is the electrosurgical coagulation electrode. The argon gas enhances the transfer of the electrical arc from the electrode to the tissues, and acts as a gaseous transport for the arc. The high flow of gas facilitates the operator as it will clear the operative field of debris and blood. The high flow rate of gas should, however, alert the surgeon to the danger of possible argon gas embolism.

Laser surgery

The development of lasers in medicine has been fast and furious. Not only are different wavelengths available to achieve differing tissue effects but the delivery systems allow the energy to be more easily applied to the tissues. The principle of current density and tissue effect in electrosurgery can be translated into laser applications. The power density of the laser beam (that is, the amount of power per unit area at the delivery site) is the equivalent to current density in laser surgery. There are, therefore, three variables to take into account when using a laser: the wavelength, the spot size and power density, and the delivery system.

The CO_2 laser operates at the far infrared spectrum of light wavelength (10 600 nm). A Helium Neon (HeNe) beam is used in conjunction with the CO_2 laser to visualize the path of the laser. This laser is usually delivered using articulated arms from source to the end of the laparoscope. The effect on the tissue is one of precise cutting and, if defocused, superficial coagulation. CO_2 laser is efficiently absorbed by water, including intracellular water, therefore the tissue effect is very localized and WYSIWYG (what you see is what you get). Often backstops are used to prevent damage beyond the area of operation. Alternatively, water may be used to submerge the operative site and thereby prevent peripheral damage. Smoke or plume evacuation is important when using a CO_2 laser so that a clear view is maintained. As a result high-flow abdominal insufflators are necessary to ensure continued pneumoperitoneum.

The Neodinium: YAG (Nd: YAG) laser operates at the near infrared range at 1064 nm. The fact that the laser is delivered via an optical fibre means that this laser can be used in the abdominal and uterine cavities with ease. It is not well absorbed by water and consequently has a deep coagulating effect. Its main use is in endometrial ablation but this laser has also been used laparoscopically. Its potential for deep coagulation must be borne in mind when operating close to vital structures, such as the ureters. Sapphire tips, attached to the end of the laser fibre, have been used to focus the Nd: YAG laser beam in an attempt to control the depth of coagulation in order to act as a cutting instrument. However, the tips are expensive and prone to falling off during operation in the abdominal cavity. Nevertheless, the fibre delivery of the Nd: YAG laser allows precise application to the tissues and the results of endometrial ablation are comparable with other methods (Garry et al 1991). Safety lies in the knowledge of the tissue effects and the working environment. A recent newcomer to the laser field is the diode laser which is a more compact and portable Nd: YAG equivalent laser. The tissue effects and capabilities are similar for both (Wyman et al 1992).

Other lasers are in use, and for the most part are fibre delivered. The argon (488–514 nm) and KTP (532 nm) lasers are in the visible range of the light spectrum. These lasers are also poorly absorbed by water but have an affinity for pigmented tissue, such as endometriosis. The pulsed Holmium: YAG (Ho: YAG) laser is a very efficient cutting instrument with little coagulation effect (Duffy et al 1992).

Other instruments

Suturing has become easier with the introduction of knot-pullers and preformed loops. In addition, small straight and curved needles may be used laparoscopically. This means effectively that any accidental damage caused during laparoscopic surgery may be initially approached through the laparoscope. However, timely recourse to laparotomy should always be considered.

Stapling devices have made the division and ligation of large pedicles possible in one move. These devices are easy to use but the tissue plains and distal extent must be clearly identified before firing to prevent division of the wrong structure. When working close to the ureters during laparoscopic surgery an illumination ureteric stent has been patented to show the lie of the ureter (Phipps & Tyrrell 1992). This device has to be inserted using a cystoscope prior to surgery.

OPERATOR ERROR

Gaining expertise in endoscopic techniques requires the operator to start with basic and simple procedures and build on this with the benefit of training. It is important to be familiar with the normal anatomy before treating the abnormal. Increasing efforts are being made to expand the role of endoscopic surgery in clinical practice, and to carry out proper evaluation. Until each indication is evaluated, cautious introduction should be the rule. Both hysteroscopy and laparoscopy have contraindications to their use and all involved in this field of gynaecology should be familiar with them.

Contraindications to hysteroscopy and laparoscopy

Hysteroscopy should not be performed in the presence of active pelvic infection. Any history of vaginal discharge or symptoms suggestive of salpingitis should be investigated first and treatment given prior to hysteroscopy. The risk to the patient is that of inducing acute endometritis or salpingitis. Cervical stenosis may make introduction of the hysteroscope difficult with the increased risk of false passage formation and even perforation. This risk may be reduced with the availability of very narrow hysteroscopes (2 mm diameter). Bleeding from the uterine cavity may result in poor vision and if it cannot be cleared easily hysteroscopy should be abandoned. However, the continuous-flow fluid-distension systems can overcome this problem. Hysteroscopy should be avoided during menstruation. The presence of cervical carcinoma is likely to lead to difficulty during hysteroscopy and if the tissue is friable and the view poor, the risk of perforation is great. Endometrial carcinoma does not mean that hysteroscopy should be avoided, as the evidence suggests that hysteroscopy does not influence disease outcome. There are few indications for hysteroscopy during pregnancy, although there was a vogue for fetoscopy in the past. If performed it should be remembered that the pregnant uterus is larger and more easily distended than the non-pregnant uterus.

Patients undergoing any form of surgery should be, if possible, medically fit. The administration of general anaesthesia has its own contraindications for which the anaesthetist should be responsible. Laparoscopy is contraindicated in a number of conditions, some of which may be categorized as relative rather than absolute. Gross obesity of the patient is a relative contra-indication to laparoscopy. An experienced operator should undertake such a case and the risks, especially of failure of pneumoperitoneum, should be explained to the patient. The presence of multiple skin incisions from previous surgery should warn the operator of the potential for underlying adhesions and distorted anatomy; again the patient should be aware of the risks of inadvertent damage, such as bowel perforation. Skin infection at the site of portal insertion is a relative contraindication. More absolute contraindications are the presence of peritonitis and bowel obstruction. Distended bowel is easily perforated by the introduction of a veress' needle or cannula. If a large abdominal or pelvic mass is present, laparoscopy is not advised. If the patient suffers from a hernia this should be corrected first as there is the possibility that the increase in abdominal pressure could lead to strangulation at the neck of the hernial sac.

Entry techniques

During hysteroscopy, the approach through the endocervical canal should be controlled and under direct vision. The use of an appropriate size of hysteroscope may be important, for example a fine hysteroscope is useful in the initial assessment of suspected Asherman's syndrome. By using the distension medium to inflate the canal and visually guiding the hysteroscope along the canal, false passages are not created and bleeding from unnecessary trauma is prevented. Some surgery requires prior dilatation of the cervix. Gentle dilatation will prevent trauma, but if there is great resistance to dilatation, to avoid laceration, a hygroscopic cervical dilator such as Dilapan™ can occasionally be useful.

Laparoscopy requires blind insufflation first, before introduction of the laparoscope. The veress' needle is best inserted at the umbilicus and the simple aspiration syringe test is a useful method of ensuring that the needle is in the right place. By aspirating, the presence of blood, urine or bowel gas will be apparent. Correct placement in the abdominal cavity will cause resistance to aspiration owing to the negative pressure. Injected air through the same syringe will be distributed into the abdominal cavity making aspiration impossible. In contrast, the pocketing effect of an extraperitoneal placement of the veress' needle will mean that air can be reaspirated after injection.

The primary portal for the laparoscope should be introduced when there is sufficient pneumoperitoneum to ensure a safe distance between the abdominal wall and underlying bowel and major vessels. Difficulty with insertion of the trocar and cannula may require widening of the skin incision in order to avoid excessive pushing, bringing the trocar too close to the posterior abdominal wall. Once the laparoscope is in place it is good practice to visualize the underlying structures to ensure no underlying damage. The extra portals used during operative laparoscopy should be sited within the safety triangle bounded by the obliterated umbilical arteries and the pubic rami, with the apex at the umbilicus. The vessels to avoid are the inferior epigastric arteries which lie lateral to the obliterated umbilical arteries. Extra portals should be sited under direct vision. Damage to the gastrointestinal tract is suspected if faecal soiling is seen or if a faecal smell is evident when changing instruments in portals or at the end of the procedure when the cannulae are removed.

Having gained access to the abdominal cavity via portal sites, when surgery is completed these sites must be secured. Failure to close defects in the rectus sheath may occasionally lead to hernia formation. Often it is necessary to place an extra suture through the defect in the sheath to ensure this complication does not occur.

Procedure-related complications

Complications during hysteroscopy depend upon the experience of the operator and the level of complexity of the surgery. Fibroid resection and the treatment of Asherman's syndrome are procedures that are more likely to have complications compared to diagnostic hysteroscopy. The more extensive the disease, the greater the expertise required. For instance, large and mainly intramural fibroids should not be tackled by a novice. Neither should the beginner attempt to treat severe Asherman's syndrome where the whole cavity has been obliterated by adhesions. Knowledge of the safety limitations set by the myometrial thickness at crucial points of the uterus (isthmus and cornua) will help reduce the risk of perforation. If perforation does occur it may be heralded by sudden loss of vision or distension. If perforation is suspected, the procedure should be stopped and the abdominal cavity inspected. The risk of intra-abdominal trauma is greatest if laser or electrosurgery were used at the time of perforation. Keeping the laser fibre or active electrode in view at all times, and always moving the activated instrument towards the operator rather than away, will reduce the risk of this complicated perforation.

Haemorrhage is avoidable if endometrial resection is confined to the superficial layers of the myometrium where the vessel diameters are relatively small (Duffy et al 1991). As intrauterine fibroids, especially those lying deep in the myometrium, often have large feeding vessels that are potential sites of haemorrhage, due care must be taken. If large vessels are opened there is also the increased risk of fluid intravasation. Intrauterine septae are usually avascular unless the line of incision penetrates too deep, with the resulting risk of haemorrhage.

Laparoscopic surgery will have risks attached to each type of surgery attempted. These complications will vary little from those encountered during their open laparotomy counterparts. General principles apply, such as exercising care when operating on the pelvic side wall, for example in the treatment of endometriosis. Underlying vital structures are at risk and precise knowledge of the local anatomy is required. All pedicles should be identified and coagulated or secured, prior to transection, in order to prevent haemorrhage. If electrosurgery is used to coagulate it should be appreciated that bipolar techniques often take longer to achieve coagulation compared to monopolar. The distal end of staple devices should be clearly seen before firing to avoid inadvertently cutting adjacent structures. Good irrigation and suction devices are essential to identify normal anatomy and sites of bleeding.

Surgical skills should be acquired gradually. By beginning with simple procedures, such as the division of fine adhesions, the endoscopic surgeon will develop the necessary hand-eye co-ordination during low-risk situations. More elaborate surgery on ectopic pregnancy and adnexectomy will form the basis before moving on to more complicated surgery. Laparoscopic hysterectomy and colposuspension will require the surgeon to be able to cope with any eventuality, and the complete skills of suturing and use of ancillary equipment are mandatory.

REFERENCES

Bosch P F 1936 Laparoscopische sterilization. Schweizerische Zeitschrift fur Krankenhaus und Anstaltswesen

Duffy S, Cobb G 1994 A practical handbook of electrosurgery. Chapman and Hall. London

Duffy S, Reid P C, Smith J H F, Sharp F 1991 In vitro studies of uterine electrosurgery. Obstet Gynecol 78: 213–220

Duffy S, Reid P C, Sharp F 1992a In vivo studies of uterine Electrosurgery. Br J Obstet Gynaecol 99: 579–582

Duffy S, Davis M, Stamp J, Sharp F 1992b Preliminary observations of Holmium:YAG laser tissue interaction using human uterus. Lasers Surg Med 12: 147–152

Garry R, Mooney P, Hasham F, Kokri M 1992 A uterine distension system to prevent fluid absorption during Nd:YAG laser endometrial ablation. Gynaecol Endosc 1: 23–29

Garry R, Erian J, Grochmal S 1991 A multicentre collaborative study into the treatment of menorrhagia by Nd:YAG laser ablation of the endometrium. Br J Obstet Gynaecol 98: 357–362

Gordon A G, Taylor P J 1993 Practical laparoscopy. Blackwell Scientific Publications, Oxford

Hope R 1937 The differential diagnosis of ectopic pregnancy by peritoneoscopy. Surg Gynaecol Obstet 64: 229–234

Hopkins H H 1953 On the diffraction theory of optical images. Proceedings of the Royal Society A217: 408

Lindemann H-J 1972 The use of CO_2 in the uterine cavity for hysteroscopy. Int J Fertil 17: 221

Magos A, Baumann R, Cheung K, Turnbull A C 1989 Intrauterine surgery during intravenous sedation as an outpatient alternative to hysterectomy. Lancet 8668: 925–926

Odell R 1993 Electrosurgery. In: Sutton C, Diamond M P (eds) Endoscopic surgery for Gynaecologists. WB Saunders, London pp 51–59

Phipps J, Tyrrell N J 1992 Transilluminating ureteric stents for preventing operative ureteric damage. Br J Obstet Gynaecol 99: 81–82

Rankin L, Steinberg L H 1992 Transcervical resection of the endometrium: a review of 400 consecutive patients. Br J Obstet Gynaecol 99: 911–914

Taylor P J, Gordon A G 1993 Practical hysteroscopy. Blackwell Scientific Publications, Oxford

Wyman A, Duffy S, Sweetland H M et al 1992 Preliminary evaluation of a new diode laser. Lasers Surg Med 12: 506–509

9

Recent advances in the diagnosis and treatment of polycystic ovary syndrome

T. J. McKenna, F. J. Hayes

Polycystic ovary syndrome, PCOS, is a condition characterized by disruption of the regular processes leading to ovulation and associated with hyperandrogenemia, normal or elevated oestrogen levels, raised LH secretion with alteration of the normal relationship between LH and FSH leading to a raised LH: FSH ratio. Macroscopically the ovaries are usually, although not always, enlarged and lobular. On histological examination the ovaries contain atretic follicles, theca cell hyperplasia and a generalized increase in stroma. On ultrasound examination the ovaries are characterized by peripheral distribution of multiple subcapsular cysts (McKenna 1992). However, the ultrasound appearances are not specific for polycystic ovary syndrome (Clayton et al 1992). Clinically PCOS presents in many patients with hirsutism and obesity in addition to oligomenorrhea. Approximately 2% of women in the general population have this syndrome and about 30% of women presenting with infertility.

PATHOGENESIS OF PCOS

The primary abnormality in PCOS could reside within the ovaries or the ovarian abnormalities could be secondary to extra-ovarian disturbances (McKenna 1988; Franks 1989; Barnes & Rosenfield 1989; Poretsky & Piper 1994). Amongst disorders of ovulation, PCOS is probably unique in that it is associated with normal or elevated oestrogen levels. This oestrogen may arise from the ovary and also peripherally mainly from fatty tissue. Thus, an abnormal oestrogen environment could feedback on gonadotrophin secretion leading to a relative excess of LH secretion compared to that of FSH, which may indeed be suppressed. This disturbance may lead to a failure of ovulation as the developing Graafian follicle depends upon stimulation from FSH. FSH stimulates the conversion of androgen to oestrogen by inducing the activity of ovarian aromatase which resides in the granulosa cell. The androgen for the granulosa cell is derived from an outer layer of theca cells in the Graafian follicle. Androgen production is controlled by LH. Where LH is excessive and FSH is suppressed this results in an imbalance leading to increased androgen production with normal or suppressed oestrogen production, principally oestradiol. Chronic

121

exposure of the ovary to this hormonal environment could lead to the development of the typical picture of PCOS.

Extensive evidence confirms that adrenal androgen excess is common in PCOS. This has been shown by means of calculated adrenal androgen production rates, and the demonstration of excessive androstenedione, DHEA and testosterone responses to stimulation by exogenous ACTH or following stimulation of endogenous ACTH secretion using metyrapone (McKenna 1988). The mechanism underlying the excess adrenal androgen production has not been established (McKenna & Cunningham 1991a). Possible mechanisms include excess stimulation of the adrenal glands by factors involved specifically in the control of androgen production. A case has been made for the existence of a specific adrenal androgen stimulating hormone (AASH). Potential candidates include β-endorphin and joining peptide. There is circumstantial *in vitro* evidence to suggest that these factors have characteristics which render them likely candidates for the AASH role (McKenna & Cunningham, in press). Alternatively, there is evidence that the metabolic clearance of cortisol is increased in PCOS. Two different sets of enzymes have been demonstrated to be excessively active in this condition, both of which are involved in the metabolism of cortisol, i.e. 5_{α}-reductase and 11β-hydroxysteroid dehydrogenase (Stewart et al 1990; Rodin et al 1994). As a consequence of increased cortisol metabolism, plasma cortisol levels will tend to fall and as a compensatory response ACTH secretion increases (Fig. 9.1). This will correct falling cortisol but

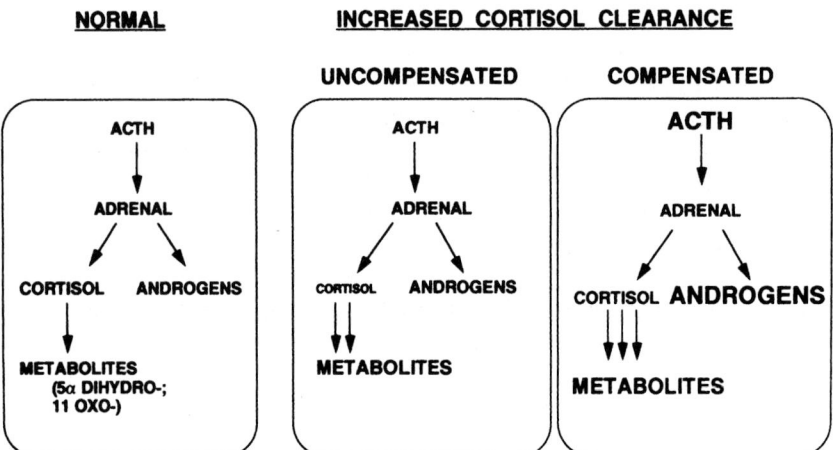

Fig. 9.1   Schematic representation of interrelationships between ACTH production from the pituitary and steroid production and metabolism from the adrenals. If cortisol metabolism is increased, peripheral cortisol levels will fall. As a consequence, a compensatory rise in ACTH secretion occurs leading to restoration of normal cortisol levels associated with a further increase in the production of cortisol metabolites and an increased production of androgens by the adrenals.

will bring about a rise in androgen levels as ACTH undoubtably plays an important, at least facilitatory, role in adrenal androgen production and secretion. An additional school of thought believes that the adrenal and ovary share a defect in the activity of the 17α-hydroxylase cytochrome P450 enzyme system. When this system is induced, there may be excess production of 17-hydroxyprogesterone and excessive conversion of 17-hydroxyprogesterone to androgens as 17–20 lyase activity is also controlled by the same enzyme (Barnes & Rosenfield 1989). Therefore, several mechanisms exist whereby adrenal androgen production may be enhanced in PCOS and supply substrate for peripheral conversion of androgen to oestrone. Oestrone may then perturb gonadotrophin secretion leading to the changes of PCOS. Alternatively, adrenal androgen excess may have a direct effect on the ovary disrupting the normal Graafian follicle development.

The primary defect in PCOS could also reside at the level of the hypothalamus-pituitary. Here, a defect in the normal mechanisms controlling gonadotrophin secretion could result in a primary derangement giving rise to the typical changes of polycystic ovaries. However, a primary abnormality residing within the pituitary-hypothalamus appears to be unlikely since gonadotrophin secretion in PCOS can be modulated or corrected by weight loss (Guzick et al 1994), by adrenal suppression (McKenna 1992) and by inhibition of oestrogen action with clomiphene treatment (Lopez-Lopez et al 1987). Another suggestion is that the primary abnormality resides in the ovary where a primary defect leads to failure of ovulation (Barnes & Rosenfield 1989) and thus to an absence of normal luteal-phase progesterone levels in the presence of normal or elevated oestrogen levels feeding back at the level of the hypothalamus-pituitary. As a consequence, abnormal LH and FSH dynamics result in the typical perturbation of gonadotrophin secretion in PCOS which leads to excess androgen production while not stimulating normal follicular development and ovulation. Recent studies have suggested that progesterone replenishment brings about a correction of gonadotrophin abnormalities and a partial lowering of elevated androgen levels (Fiad et al 1993).

It is certainly possible that there is no one specific initiating factor in patients with primary PCOS. Rather, PCOS may represent a common endpoint for any mechanism bringing about ovulation arrest in the presence of oestrogen levels which are not suppressed. In addition to an intrinsic ovarian abnormality other potential initiating abnormalities include excess adrenal androgen secretion, obesity and hyperinsulinemia usually associated with insulin resistance (Fig. 9.2).

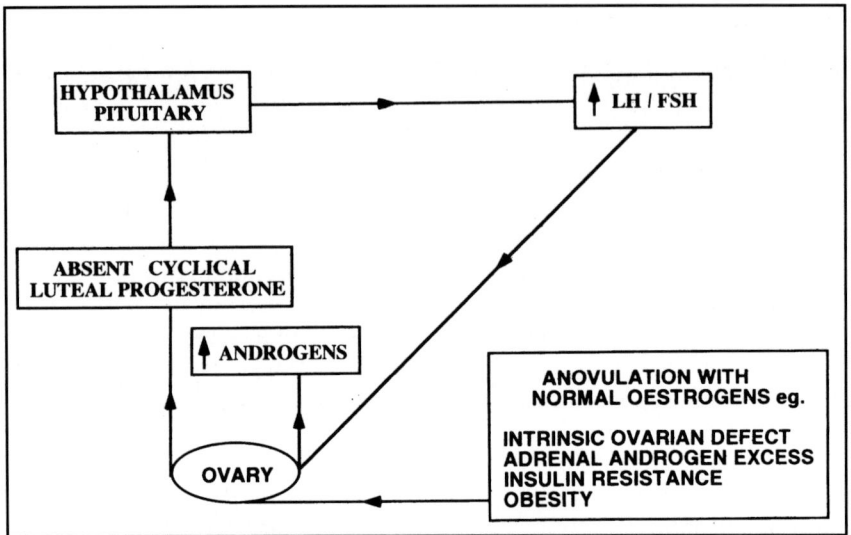

Fig. 9.2   Schematic representation of model for the development of PCOS. It is proposed that when anovulation occurs in association with normal or elevated oestrogen levels, irrespective of the cause, the absence of normal cyclical luteal-phase progesterone levels brings about excess LH secretion and an increase in the LH to FSH ratio. As a result of this, ovarian androgen secretion increases and the processes of Graafian follicle maturation leading to ovulation are inhibited further.

DIAGNOSIS

Clinical features

Polycystic ovary syndrome has a gradual onset in young women who typically first become aware of a few excess hairs which may be present on the upper lip, chin, neck, periareolar areas, lower abdomen or upper thighs and the arms may also be affected. Hirsutism progresses slowly and usually does not come to medical attention for at least 1 year after it was first noted. The onset of symptoms is typically in the decade between 15 and 25 years. Some women with PCOS do not manifest hirsutism and this may represent a degree of androgen resistance. Acne is frequently present in addition to hirsutism. Women with PCOS tend to be obese. Evidence of frank virilization such as temporal recession of the hairline, deepening of the voice, increase in muscle mass or clitoromegaly does not occur in PCOS. Amenorrhea or an irregular menstrual pattern may be the presenting symptom. Some women with PCOS have irregular but frequent menstruation, which on evaluation, is not usually associated with ovulation. These women may present with PCOS when they fail to become pregnant. In addition to reduced conception, pregnancy outcome may also be adversely affected with miscarriage rates as high as 65% being reported (Regan et al 1990).

Differential diagnoses

The differential diagnosis of hirsutism and oligomenorrhea includes congenital adrenal hyperplasia, Cushing's syndrome, benign and malignant androgen-secreting tumours of the adrenals or ovaries and hyperthecosis ovarii (McKenna 1992; McKenna 1994). The major features which distinguish these disorders are outlined in Table 9.1.

Table 9.1   Differential diagnosis of hirsutism and oligomenorrhoea based on clinical and hormonal features

	Polycystic ovary syndrome	Congenital[a] adrenal hyperplasia	Cushing's syndrome	Androgen-secreting tumours	Hyperthecosis ovarii
Time of onset	15–25 years	Congenital	Any time	Any time	Any time
Time of onset to medical presentation	Years	May present at birth, adolescence, or childhood	Months to Years	Weeks to Months	Years
Virilization	Rare	+	Unusual	+	+
Clinical comment	Obesity (40%)	Short stature, labial fusion, primary amenorrhoea	Evidence of glucocorticoid excess	Mass may be palpable	
Testosterone	↑in 75%	↑↑*	N/↑	↑↑	↑↑
17-OH Progesterone	N/↑	↑↑*	N/↑[#]	N/↑[#]	N/↑
Cortisol post-dexamethasone	Suppressed	Suppressed	Not suppressed	Ovarian: suppressed Adrenal: not suppressed	Suppressed
Luteinizing hormone	↑	N/↑	N/↑	↓	N
Follicle stimulating hormone	↓	N/↓	N/↓	↓	N

+, Present; –, absent; ↑, elevated; ↓ , decreased.* Suppresses on treatment with replacement doses of glucocorticoid taken at night; #progesterone and other precursors e.g. 11-deoxycortisol, 17-OH-pregnenolone may be elevated in patients with an adrenal carcinoma; [a]congenital adrenal hyperplasia represented here is of the 21-hydroxylase deficiency type only.

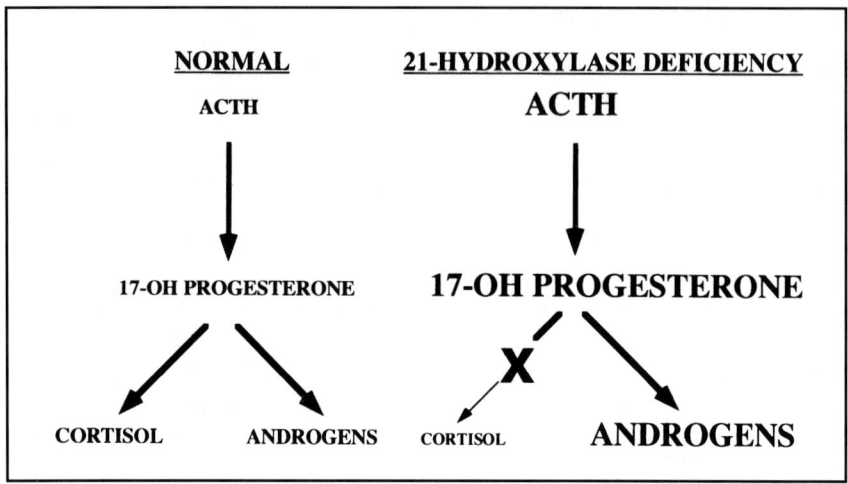

Fig. 9.3   Schematic representation of the steroidogenic consequences of 21-hydroxylase deficiency. The conversion of 17-hydroxyprogesterone to cortisol is dependent upon the enzyme 21-hydroxylase. The conversion of 17-hydroxyprogesterone to androgens is not dependent upon 21-hydroxylation. In the presence of 21-hydroxylase deficiency cortisol levels fall and 17-hydroxyprogesterone, the substrate of 21-hydroxylase, accumulates. In attempting to bring plasma cortisol levels into the normal range, ACTH secretion increases. Correction of cortisol deficiency is associated with excessive stimulation of the normally functioning androgen-producing pathway which leads to the development of hyperandrogenemia with its clinical consequences.

Congenital adrenal hyperplasia is a broad term which covers a number of defects in the steroid biosynthetic pathway leading to cortisol production. The most frequently occurring form of congenital adrenal hyperplasia is 21-hydroxylase deficiency. In this disorder 17-hydroxyprogesterone accumulates and cortisol levels fall causing ACTH levels to rise, and since 21-hydroxylase deficiency does not reduce androgen production, adrenal androgen hypersecretion results (Fig. 9.3). Two distinct congenital disorders give rise to 21-hydroxylase deficiency (Miller 1991). The more severe disorder usually presents soon after birth with evidence of adrenal insufficiency and ambiguous genitalia in affected females. However, there is a milder, distinct genetic abnormality giving rise to 21-hydroxylase deficiency which may become apparent in early adulthood or may go undetected i.e. late onset and cryptic forms respectively (New 1992). The frequency with which the milder form of congenital adrenal hyperplasia may be found in patients presenting with features typical of PCOS varies from less than 1% to approximately 30% depending on the communities examined. In Mediterranean races, the frequency may be approximately 10% while in Northern Europeans the frequency of congenital adrenal hyperplasia in the general population is low and the likelihood of a patient presenting with typical features of PCOS having underlying congenital adrenal hyperplasia is less than 1%. Affected members tend to grow rapidly in childhood but to stop growing earlier than normal so that the tall child becomes a small adult.

Cushing's syndrome, glucocorticoid excess of any aetiology, is frequently associated with androgen excess though this may be relatively mild. Cushing's syndrome may be caused by pituitary ACTH excess, benign or malignant adrenal tumours and ectopic ACTH production. In Cushing's disease, pituitary ACTH excess, the development of hirsutism and menstrual irregularities may progress rapidly and may occur at any age but virilization is rare. However, there are striking features of glucocorticoid excess. Ectopic ACTH production is also associated with very variable androgen levels from subnormal to markedly excessive (Cunningham & McKenna 1994). The condition is usually rapidly progressive and may be associated with muscle wasting and hypokalaemia while the responsible tumour which elaborates ACTH may be undetected. Such tumours are most frequently located in the thorax (small cell tumours and carcinoids), and pancreas.

Patients with adrenal or ovarian androgen-secreting tumours may present at any age, give a history of rapid progression of symptoms and signs and they may demonstrate evidence of virilization (Freedman 1991). Localizing procedures, including CT scanning of the adrenals and ultrasound examination of the ovaries, are frequently sufficient to identify the presence of the tumour. Malignant tumours tend to be large and metastasize early.

Hyperthecosis ovarii is a benign disorder of the ovaries which may be a severe extension of PCOS but is more likely to be a distinct disorder in its own right. It is characterized histologically by the presence of nests of luteinized theca cells in a hyperplastic ovarian stroma and is manifest clinically as masculinization and menstrual disturbances, which may occur at any age (Nagamani et al 1981). Hyperthecosis should be suspected in any patient who presents with severe hyperandrogenemia in the absence of evidence of Cushing's syndrome, congenital adrenal hyperplasia or an adrenal or ovarian tumour. While there is considerable clinical overlap with PCOS, patients with hyperthecosis differ in that they tend to be virilized as well as severely hirsute and while morphologically the ovaries are enlarged, they are not typically polycystic. Many patients ultimately require bilateral oophorectomy to halt progressive virilization.

THE INVESTIGATION OF THE HIRSUTE/ OLIGOMENORRHOEIC PATIENT

Since greater than 95% of patients presenting in Northern Europe with hirsutism have the relatively benign conditions of idiopathic hirsutism (hirsutism associated with regular ovulation) or typical PCOS, and approximately 5% of the general population are hirsute, a major opportunity for excessive laboratory and imaging investigation exists for the unwary

(McKenna 1994). The vast majority of patients with PCOS conform to a highly specific clinical presentation seldom shared by other disorders (Table 9.1). Where features atypical of PCOS exist, additional investigations are warranted. These should include specific procedures to examine for the presence of congenital adrenal hyperplasia, androgen-secreting tumours of the adrenals and ovaries, and Cushing's syndrome. Screening for congenital adrenal hyperplasia is particularly indicated in those populations in which the disorder is known to have a high prevalence, including Mediterranean races and specific groups with a very high prevalence of 21-hydroxylase deficiency e.g. Askenasi Jews and Eskimos. Measurement of 17-hydroxyprogesterone in early-morning blood samples will usually identify the affected individuals. Screening can also be conducted at any time by examining the 17-hydroxyprogesterone response to adrenal stimulation using 1–24 ACTH, 250 µg IV. Dr New and her colleagues have devised a nomogram which allows identification of affected individuals (Miller 1991; New

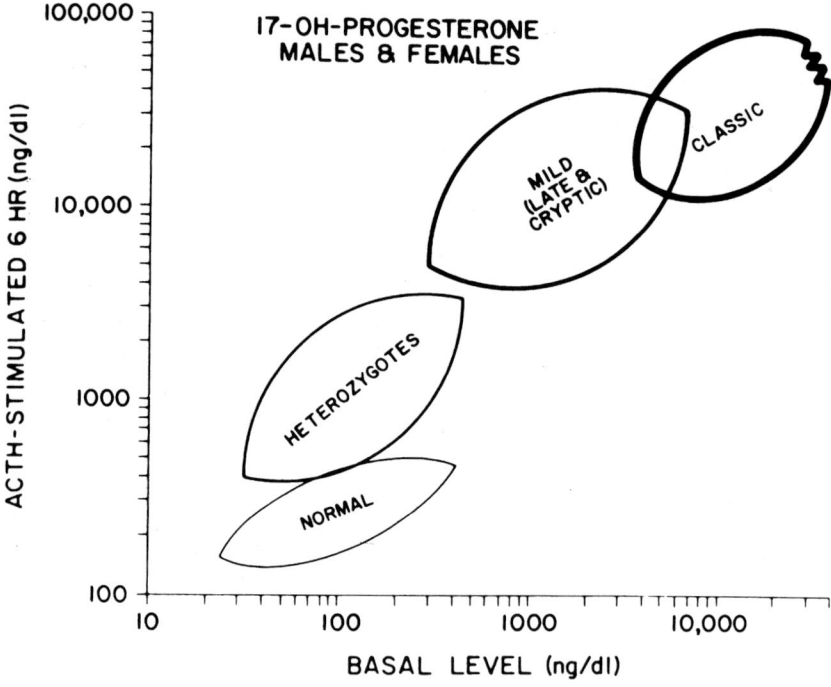

Fig. 9.4 This nomogram has been derived from careful analysis of the relationship between basal and ACTH-stimulated 17-hydroxyprogesterone levels in a group of subjects who have been specifically classified according to whether they are: homozygous for the classical 21-hydroxylase deficiency gene defect, homozygous for the late onset 21-hydroxylase gene defect, heterozygous for these defects, i.e. unaffected carriers, or homozygous for not carrying the defect, i.e. unaffected non-carriers designated 'normal'. Reprinted from Rosenfield & Miller 1983 with permission of the Publishers John Wright, PSG Inc, Bristol.

1992). Figure 9.4 is redrawn from their data to outline schematically the information which can be derived from the ACTH test when combined with careful genetic analysis.

The presence of adrenal tumours, which is suggested by very high androgen levels found in patients with rapidly progressing symptoms and evidence of virilization, can be confirmed if a characteristic lesion is identified on imaging procedures of the adrenals and ovaries (Freedman 1991). DHEAS, androstenedione and 11-deoxycortisol are frequently found to be markedly elevated. The finding of an elevated DHEAS level acts as a marker for adrenal involvement. However, adrenal tumours may be present in the absence of elevated DHEAS (McKenna et al 1990). Should imaging procedures fail to localize a tumour in a patient where the suspicion is high, catheterization of adrenal and ovarian veins may be undertaken. In some patients, laparotomy may be required to examine the adrenals and ovaries where the tumour is small and other localizing procedures have proved ineffective.

TREATMENT

General measures

Weight loss.   Obesity is a frequent component of PCOS. Whether this is aetiologically important or whether obesity occurs as a consequence of hyperinsulinaemia, is uncertain. However, for many patients weight loss is associated with normalization of the hormonal disturbances and the resumption of regular ovulation (Guzick et al 1994). Certainly, the general beneficial effects of weight loss with PCOS probably extend beyond the question of infertility. Patients with PCOS have a high prevalence of abnormal glucose tolerance and probably carry a high risk for cardiovascular disease (Conway & Jacobs 1993). Weight loss will have a beneficial impact on these consequences of PCOS.

Cigarette smoking.   A number of studies have suggested that in some way cigarette smoking may stimulate adrenal androgens. Postmenopausal women who smoke have higher DHEAS levels than postmenopausal women who do not smoke. Furthermore, in premenopausal hirsute women androstenedione levels were significantly higher amongst smokers than in women who did not smoke (Byrne et al 1991).

Treatment of hirsutism

Hormonal measures

Oestrogen.   For patients who wish to obtain hormonal treatment and who do not wish to become pregnant, treatment with oestrogen is the mainstay. The effect of oestrogen is to suppress gonadotrophin secretion, suppress ovarian androgen secretion, and suppress adrenal steroid bio-synthesis (Givens 1983). The much-reported effect of oestrogen on sex-hormone binding globulin is probably an epiphenomenon and does not contribute to the lowering of peripheral free testosterone levels in blood. Changes in protein-binding capacity will lead to a resetting of total androgen levels but will have little, if any, effect on the free androgen levels as long as testosterone production and metabolic clearance rates remain unchanged. A change in protein-binding levels will be associated with a short-lived change in free levels until a new steady state has been established. None-theless, oestrogen achieves marked suppression in androgen production (ovarian and adrenal) resulting in extremely low free testosterone levels which reach sub-physiological values in most patients (McKenna & Cunningham 1991b). The combination of oestrogen with a non-androgenic progestogen is an effective form of treatment for hirsutism if maintained for adequate duration. The hair growth cycle has recently been comprehensively reviewed (Randall 1994). If suppression of androgen levels is associated with abolition of stimulation to new hair growth and the slowing down of existing hair growth, it will take a minimum of 2 years under optimal conditions to achieve a clearing of hirsutism. The best treatment results are achieved by supplementing hormonal with cosmetic measures during this time.

Anti-androgens.   Cyproterone acetate has been the most widely used anti-androgen in the treatment of hirsutism. This is an effective anti-androgen and has been used successfully to block male androgen levels. Traditionally this agent has been used in the reverse sequential method. Because cyproterone acetate has a long half-life, in order to ensure regular withdrawal bleeding when it is given in combination with oestrogen, cyproterone acetate is prescribed for the first 10 days of a 21-day course of oestrogen. Oestrogen is then interrupted for 7 days during which withdrawal bleeding occurs and the cycle is repeated. Good results were reported with this combination using doses of cyproterone acetate 50–100 mg daily, but some patients experienced side effects which included breast discomfort, weight gain and lack of libido. A recent study has compared effects on hirsutism of using a constant level of oestrogen in combination with 2, 25 or 100 mg of cyproterone acetate. There was no significant difference be-tween the beneficial effects achieved (Barth et al 1991). This is hardly surprising when one considers that the amount of free testosterone available during treatment with oestrogen is sub-physiological and it will take little anti-androgen to block its effect. Oestrogen has been used in combination with the anti-androgen in order to ensure effective contraception. Exposure of a male fetus to anti-androgen will result in feminization of the external genitalia. Low-dose cyproterone acetate, 2 mg daily for a 21-day cycle is combined with ethinyl oestradiol, 35 µg, in a commonly prescribed pre-paration which is not associated with delay of withdrawal bleeding and is effective in providing an improvement of approximately 50% in the Ferriman-Gallwey scoring system for hirsutism, over 6–9 months (McKenna & Cunningham 1991b). While some authors claim an improved response using higher doses of cyproterone acetate, the only controlled study does not support this and the practice does not have a rational basis.

Alternative anti-androgens include spironolactone, a drug initially used for its mineralocorticoid antagonist properties. This is the agent used most widely as an anti-androgen in the United States, where cyproterone acetate has not been approved for the treatment of hirsutism (Barth et al 1989). Spironolactone is usually used continuously and generally with an anovulant in women of reproductive age because of the concern of damage to the developing fetus if present in a women receiving anti-androgen. Spironolactone 50–100 mg per day, is frequently associated with menstrual irregularities. It has the advantage of being an agent which is particularly useful in the treatment of hypertensive women or in women who exhibit hypertension when treated with oestrogen. It is unusual for electrolyte disturbances to develop but patients should be monitored for the development of postural hypotension, hyperkalaemia or hyponatraemia.

Adrenal suppression.   Adrenal androgen excess is common in women with PCOS and idiopathic hirsutism. Treatment with physiological doses of glucocorticoid given at midnight, to inhibit the early morning surge in ACTH secretion and thus glucocorticoid and androgen secretion, has been used for hirsute women. Dexamethasone 0.25–0.5 mg or prednisone 5–7.5 mg at midnight or when retiring, has proven to be very successful in the suppression of androgen levels, correction of gonadotrophin secretion, resumption of regular menstruation in women with PCOS and in achieving a significant decrease in hirsutism by 6 months in approximately 40% of affected women (Loughlin et al 1986). Adrenal suppression is unique amongst the treatments of hirsutism, as it facilitates ovulation. All other forms of treatment are associated with ovarian suppression, or are treatments where pregnancy is contraindicated e.g. anti-androgens. However, treatment of obese women with dexamethasone is frequently associated with further weight gain. It appears that obese women are particularly sensitive to the appetite-stimulating properties of glucocorticoids.

Miscellaneous.   A variety of treatments for hirsutism has been suggested from time-to-time but they are not of proven efficacy, or have disadvantages in the terms of side effects or of treatment complexity so that they do not present a reasonable alternative to oestrogens, conventional anti-androgens or adrenal suppression. These agents included drugs that inhibit 5α-reductase activity, which is responsible for the conversion of testosterone to 5α-dihydrotestosterone, the biologically active androgen in the hair follicle (Brooks 1986).

Cosmetic measures

In order to obtain an acceptable short-term cosmetic result, local measures are essential. The widely held view that removal of hair stimulates stronger growth and encourages spread has little to substantiate it. Patients should be encouraged to use cosmetic measures alone for non-androgen-dependent hair and to supplement hormonal treatment with local measures for patients with excess androgen-dependent hair growth. While the hair growth will return following plucking, use of depilatory creams or waxing, the procedures may be repeated. Should a particular form of treatment cause skin irritation, alternative treatments or other preparations of similar treatment (e.g. depilatory creams) should be used until a compatible treatment is identified. For some patients, particularly those with fine, dark hair in the sideburn and upper lip regions, bleaching gives the best results. Should the advised bleaching mixture cause burning, modifications can be tried particularly on less sensitive skin, e.g. back of the hand. Of the local measures available only electrolysis, when performed properly, gives a good long-term result. Clinicians who undertake the treatment of hirsutism should identify a reputable electrolysist for their patients. Clinicians should also ensure that patients have reasonable expectations and encourage patients to use local measures as a supplement to hormonal treatment with the anticipation that the frequency of need for cosmetic measures will decrease as the duration of hormonal treatment increases.

Treatment of infertility

Since PCOS accounts for approximately 25–30% of infertility in women and approximately 15% of overall infertility, the treatment of this condition is of both medical and social importance. Treatments used include anti-oestrogens, adrenal suppression, gonadotrophin treatment, gonadotrophin-releasing hormone (GnRH), GnRH analogues, ovarian wedge resection and electrocautery.

Medical therapy

Anti-oestrogen. Inhibition of oestrogen feedback at the level of hypothalamus-pituitary has been associated with a surge in FSH secretion. This surge in FSH secretion is associated with growth of the Graafian follicle and an increase in oestrogen secretion. When successful the Graafian follicle continues to enlarge and eventually ruptures releasing an ovum i.e. ovulation. Approximately 80% of PCOS women treated with clomiphene citrate ovulate and approximately 40% become pregnant (Kelly & Adashi 1987). However, there is a high miscarriage rate of approximately 40%, which may be a result of the abnormal hormonal milieu e.g. high androgen levels present in the PCOS patient. Pretreatment of patients with a progestogen e.g. medroxyprogesterone acetate, has been associated with an increased frequency of ovulation induction in patients subsequently treated with an anti-oestrogen e.g. clomiphene citrate (Homburg et al 1988). Clomiphene is usually given in a dose of 50 mg daily for 5 days. If menstrual bleeding has not occurred within 6 weeks of administration of this agent, a pregnancy test should be performed. If the pregnancy test proves to be negative, then retreatment with clomiphene citrate at a higher dose, 100 mg daily, should be undertaken. The dose may be increased by 50 mg increments to 200 mg until ovulation is achieved. Ovarian hyperstimulation can arise with clomiphene in the patient with PCOS. Where a dose of clomiphene citrate is found to be successful in the induction of ovulation, this dose should be repeated for 6 treatment cycles or until pregnancy is achieved. The monitoring of ovulation should consist of clinical evaluation including history of the menstrual characteristics. Ovulation can be confirmed by the finding of progesterone levels typical of the mid-luteal phase of the menstrual cycle approximately 1 week prior to the next anticipated menstrual bleed. Clomiphene citrate is associated with a higher than normal incidence of multiple births i.e. approximately 10% of clomiphene-induced pregnancies will be associated with twins and approximately 1% with 3 or more babies (Kelly & Adashi 1987).

High-dose clomiphene citrate treatment associated with Graafian follicle stimulation may also be associated with the development of large ovarian cysts and ovarian hyperstimulation syndrome (Blacker 1992). This condition is characterized by an increased vascular permeability which is thought to be prostaglandin mediated, resulting in a shift of body fluid from the intravascular to the extravascular compartments (Borenstein 1989). This is associated with the development of ascites, pleural effusion and hypovolaemic shock. Patients who develop this condition should be treated with plasma expanders. The role of prostaglandin synthetase inhibitors is a matter of debate. Abdominal paracentesis should be reserved for the relief of dyspnoea and abdominal discomfort in patients with severe hyperstimulation syndrome and should only be performed under ultrasound guidance. Full-length TED stockings are recommended to reduce the risk of venous thrombosis. Untreated patients may progress to irreversible shock and death. Abdominal discomfort in patients on ovulation induction programmes should be taken as a warning signal for the possible development of hyperstimulation syndrome. Under these circumstances treatment should be interrupted, blood obtained for measurement of oestrogen levels and ultrasound examination of the ovaries performed. Hyperstimulation is usually associated with the presence of several large ovarian cysts i.e. greater than 20 mm in diameter, and free fluid in the abdomen. Oestrogen levels are usually in excess of 5 500 pmol/L. In patients undergoing prolonged clomiphene citrate treatment using doses in excess of 100 mg daily, ultrasound monitoring is recommended to determine the number of follicles developing. Graafian follicles or ovarian cysts in excess of 20 mm in diameter, constitute warning signals that ovarian hyperstimulation syndrome may evolve if treatment is continued.

Adrenal suppression.   Approximately 60% of PCOS patients treated with glucocorticoid resume regular ovulation (Loughlin et al 1986). This is associated with an improvement in the hormonal status and theoretically should be associated with an improved pregnancy rate and a lower miscarriage rate. Steinberger and colleagues (1981) treated a large group of patients and reported an outcome similar to that associated with clomiphene citrate. However, adrenal suppression does not appear to be associated with an increased incidence of multiple pregnancies or with the development of hyperstimulation syndrome. Treatment with dexamethasone is simple i.e. 0.25–0.5 mg each night, and does not require specific intervention to stimulate ovulation (Loughlin et al 1986). This form of treatment also brings about an improvement in hirsutism and acne because of its androgen-lowering effects. Combination treatment of dexamethasone with clomiphene citrate is associated with a higher rate of ovulation induction than is achieved with either treatment used alone (Fayez 1976).

Gonadotrophin therapy.   Human menopausal gonadotrophins are potent ovulation-inducing agents, indicated for PCOS patients who fail to conceive in response to clomiphene citrate. Available preparations consist of a combination of LH and FSH (Pergonal) or purified FSH which are equipotent (Ginsburg & Hardiman 1991). Exogenously administered gonadotrophins stimulate the ovary directly resulting in follicular maturation, and human chorionic gonadotrophin (hCG), which functions as a surrogate luteinizing hormone, is then required to trigger release of the mature ovum. Because of the significant risk of ovarian hyperstimulation syndrome and multiple pregnancy associated with gonadotrophin therapy, specialist supervision and close monitoring is mandatory. This requires both daily oestradiol measurements and alternate-day ovarian ultrasound examination. Because sensitivity to gonadotrophins may vary, the dose must be titrated according to the response of the individual patient. Treatment may be commenced using FSH 75U and increased by 75U every 3 days if oestradiol levels have not doubled or follicle size is not increasing (Blacker 1992). Once follicle size is 15–18 mm, hCG 5 000 U should be administered. Treatment with hCG should be withheld if oestradiol levels exceed 5500 pmol/L, if more than 4 dominant follicles are present, or if follicle size is greater than 18 mm. Following these guidelines the risk of significant ovarian hyperstimulation is minimized. The risk of multiple pregnancy correlates with the number of dominant follicles present at the timing of hCG administration, so that it is approximately 4% when 2 dominant follicles are present, increasing to 18% in the presence of 3–4 dominant follicles (Kelly & Adashi 1987). The pregnancy rate for gonadotrophin therapy in clomiphene-resistant PCOS is approximately 20%. This low success rate may reflect release of endogenous gonadotrophins from the pituitary in response to rising oestrogen levels leading to an early LH surge before the follicles reach maturity. Pretreatment with a GnRH agonist to prevent premature luteinization has been associated with a higher conception rate (Dodson et al 1987).

The incidence of spontaneous miscarriage following gonadotrophin therapy may be as high as 30% (Ginsburg & Hardiman 1991). In an effort to overcome the problems associated with conventional gonadotrophin therapy in PCOS, namely the low pregnancy rate and increased risk of miscarriage, multiple pregnancy and ovarian hyperstimulation, alternative gonadotrophin regimens, have been proposed. Franks and Hamilton-Fairley (in press) advocate the use of low-dose gonadotrophins with a starting dose of 52.5 IU, which may be maintained for up to 14 days. A variation of the low-dose regimen, the so-called step down protocol, has recently been proposed and attempts to mimic the FSH profile seen in natural cycles. In this protocol, which starts with a conventional high dose of gonado-trophin, the dose is gradually reduced as follicles develop. Following the low-dose regimen the incidence of multiple pregnancy was only 7% and there were no cases of severe hyperstimulation syndrome. However, the pregnancy and miscarriage rates were disappointingly similar to those ob-served with conventional-dose gonadotrophin therapy.

Gonadotrophin-Releasing Hormone. Gonadotrophin-Releasing Hor-mone (GnRH) is a decapeptide first isolated, sequenced and synthesized in 1971. Its clinical efficacy is dependent on pulsatile administration deliv-ered either subcutaneously (SC) or intravenously (IV) by a small portable programmable infusion pump. In studies in which the two methods of administration have been compared, the IV route was found to be more effective and patients resistant to SC pulsatile GnRH frequently responded to IV therapy. The usual dose is 5–10 μg IV or 10–20 μg SC administered in pulses every 60–90 minutes. Martin et al (1990) recommend a 90 minute interval for the first week of folliculogenesis, increasing to 60 minutes in the mid-follicular phase until ovulation occurs. The frequency of GnRH administration is then slowed to every 90 minutes for 1 week after ovulation and thereafter to every 4 hours for the remainder of the luteal phase until either menstruation or pregnancy ensues. As an alternative to continuing GnRH therapy, luteal phase support may be provided by administering hCG 2000 U every 3rd day over 6 days. The ovulatory rate achieved with pulsatile GnRH therapy in PCOS does generally not exceed 40–50%, with a pregnancy rate of approximately 16% per cycle (Filicori et al 1991). How-ever, treatment with a GnRH analogue for 6–8 weeks prior to the initiation of pulsatile GnRH therapy, which has the effect of lowering both intraovarian androgens and the LH: FSH ratio, increases the ovulatory rate to approxi-mately 80% and the pregnancy rate to approximately 30%. Because endog-enous feedback mechanisms are still operative during pulsatile GnRH therapy, the degree of monitoring required is considerably less than for gonadotrophin therapy. In addition, the incidence of multiple pregnancy is lower at 5–8% and significant ovarian hyperstimulation has never been reported (Martin et al 1990).

Surgical therapy

While wedge resection of the ovaries is no longer used as a treatment option, electrocautery of the ovaries has been introduced. The mechanism, whereby cauterization of cystic areas through the external surface of the ovaries is associated with a decline in testosterone and LH levels and an increase in FSH levels, resumption of ovulation and the occurrence of pregnancy is not understood but well documented (Abdel Gadir et al 1990). The miscarriage rate associated with pregnancy following electrocautery was similar to that of pregnancies occurring following gonadotrophin treatment. In addition, patients who failed to resume ovulation following electrocautery were more responsive to clomiphene treatment after the procedure than they had been prior to electrocautery. This form of therapy expands the options available but may result in tubo-ovarian adhesions. It may prove to be useful for patients resistant to medical treatment, when medical treatment is contraindicated e.g. patients demonstrating hyperstimulation syndrome in response to conventional therapy, or where fiscal constraints preclude the availability of gonadotrophins etc.

KEY POINTS FOR CLINICAL PRACTICE

1. Greater than 95% of patients presenting with hirsutism and oligomenorrhea have PCOS.

2. Features that suggest a disorder other than PCOS include onset of symptoms outside the decade 15–25 years, rapid progression, the presence of virilization (balding, clitoromegaly, increased muscle mass, deepening of the voice), features of Cushing's syndrome.

3. Disorders other than PCOS which present with hirsutism and oligomenorrhea include congenital adrenal hyperplasia, Cushing's syndrome, hyperthecosis ovarii, and adrenal and ovarian androgen-secreting benign and malignant tumours (see Table 9.1).

4. Oestrogen with a non-androgenic progestogen and antiandrogens are the most effective treatment agents for hirsutism.

5. Alternative treatments include glucocorticoids when continued ovulation is desired and spironolactone for hypertensive patients.

6. Local cosmetic measures are important in the management of hirsutism.

7. Clomiphene citrate is the first choice agent for ovulation induction. Glucocorticoid treatment is probably underused and the combination of clomiphene citrate and glucocorticoid or progestagen is more successful than these agents used alone.

8. Clomiphene-resistant patients may respond to gonadotrophin treatment used conventionally, in low dose, in a step-down regimen or following treatment with Gn-RH analogues.

9. Electrocautery of the ovaries is useful for patients for whom medical treatment is unsuccessful or may not be available.

REFERENCES

Abdel Gadir A, Mowafi R S, Alnaser H M I et al 1990 Laparoscopic ovarian electrocautery versus human menopausal gonadotrophins and pure follicle-stimulating hormone in the treatment of patients with polycystic ovary syndrome. Clin Endocrinol (Oxf) 33: 585–592

Barnes R, Rosenfield R L 1989 The polycystic ovary syndrome: pathogenesis and treatment. Ann Intern Med 101: 386–399

Barth J H, Cherry C A, Wojnarowska F, Dawber R P R 1989 Spironolactone is an effective and well-tolerated systemic anti-androgen therapy for hirsute women. J Clin Endocrinol Metab 68: 966–970

Barth J H, Cherry C A, Wojnarowska F, Dawber R P R 1991 Cyproterone acetate for severe hirsutism: results of a double-blind dose-ranging study. Clin Endocrinol (Oxf) 35: 5–10

Blacker C M 1992 Ovulation stimulation and induction. Endo Metab Clin N Amer 21: 68–73

Borenstein R, Elholah U, Lunenfeld B, Schwartz Z S 1989 Severe ovarian hyperstimulation syndrome: a re-evaluated therapeutic approach. Fertil Steril 51: 791–795.

Brooks J R 1986 Treatment of hirsutism with 5α-reductase inhibitors. Clin Endocrinol Metab 15: 391–405

Byrne B, Cunningham S K, Igoe D et al 1991 Sex steroids, adiposity and smoking in the pathogenesis of idiopathic hirsutism and PCOS Acta Endocrinol (Copenhagen) 124: 370–374

Clayton R N, Ogden V, Hodgkinson C et al 1992 How common are polycystic ovaries in normal women and what is their significance for the fertility of the population? Clin Endocrinol (Oxf) 37: 127–134

Conway G S, Jacobs H S, 1993 Clinical implications of hyperinsulinaemia in women. Clin Endocrinol (Oxf) 39: 623–632

Cunningham S K, McKenna T J 1994 Dissociation of adrenal androgen and cortisol secretion in Cushing's syndrome. Clin Endocrinol (Oxf) 41: 795–800

Dodson W C, Hughes C I, Whiteslider D B, Haney A F 1987 The effect of leuprolide acetate on ovulation induction with human menopausal gonadotrophins in polycystic ovary syndrome. J Clin Endocrinol Metab 65: 95–100

Fayez J A 1976 Selection of patients for clomiphene citrate therapy. Obstet Gynecol 47: 671–676

Fiad T M, Culhton M, Dunbar J et al 1993 Gonadotrophin, androgen and oestrogen abnormalities in polycystic ovary syndrome occurs secondary to anovulation and progesterone deficiency. J Endocrinol(Suppl) 139: 32

Filicori M, Flamigni C, Merrigiola M C et al 1991 Ovulation induction with pulsatile gonadotrophin-releasing hormone: technical modalities and clinical perspectives. Fertil Steril 56: 1–13

Franks S 1989 Polycystic ovary syndrome: changing prospective. Clin Endocrinol 31: 87–120.

Franks S, Hamilton-Fairley D Ovulation induction: gonadotrophins. In: Adashi E Y, Rock J A, Rosenwaks Z (eds) Reproductive Endocrinology, Surgery, Technology. Raven Press, New York, (in press).

Freedman D A 1991 Steroid hormone-producing tumours of the adrenal, ovary and testes Endocrinol Metab Clin N Amer 20: 751–766

Ginsburg J, Hardiman P 1991 The response to gonadotrophin therapy in infertile women with polycystic ovaries. In: Shaw R W (ed) Polycystic ovaries–a disorder or symptom? Parthenon Publishing Company, New Jersey, pp 165–178

Givens J R 1983 Role of oral contraceptives in the treatment of hyperandrogenism of hirsute women In: Mahesh V V, Greenblatt R B (eds) Hirsutism and virilism: pathogenesis, diagnosis and management. John Wright/PSG, Boston, MA. pp 351–367

Guzick D S, Wing R, Smith D et al 1994 Endocrine consequences of weight loss in obese hyperandrogenic anovulatory women Fertil Steril 61: 598–604

Homburg R, Weissglas L, Goldman J 1988 Improved treatment of anovulation in polycystic ovarian disease utilizing the effect of progesterone on the inappropriate gonadotrophin release and clomiphene response. Human Reproduction 3: 285–288

Kelly J L, Adashi E Y 1987 Ovulation induction. Obstet Gynecol Clin North Amer 14: 831

Lopez-Lopez E, Noguera M C, Fuente T et al 1987 Response to clomiphene citrate in polycystic ovarian syndrome according to different LH: FSH ratios. Hum Reprod 2: 635–638

Loughlin T, Cunningham S, Moore A et al 1986 Adrenal abnormalities in polycystic ovary syndrome. J Clin Endocrinol Metab 62: 142–147

Martin K, Santoro N, Hall J et al 1990 Management of ovulatory disorders with pulsatile gonadotrophin-releasing hormone. J Clin Endocrinol Metab, Clinical Review Series 71: 1018A–1018G

McKenna T J 1988 Pathogenesis and treatment of polycystic ovary syndrome. N Engl J Med 318: 558–562

McKenna T J 1992 Hirsutism and Polycystic Ovary Syndrome. In: Grossman A (ed) Clinical Endocrinology. Blackwell Scientific Publications, London, pp 691–712

McKenna T J 1994 Screening for sinister causes of hirsutism N Engl J Med 331: 1015–1016

McKenna T J, Cunningham S K 1991a The control of adrenal androgen secretion. J Endocrinol 129: 1–3

McKenna T J, Cunningham S K, 1991b Role for a non-androgenic anovulant in the management of hirsutism. Irish J Med Sci 160: 194–196

McKenna T J, Cunningham S K Adrenal androgen production in women with hirsutism. Eur J Endocrinol (In press)

McKenna T J, O'Connell Y, Cunningham S et al 1990 Steroidogenesis in an oestrogen-producing adrenal tumour in a young woman: comparison with steroid profiles associated with cortisol and androgen-producing tumours. J Clin Endocrinol Metab 70: 28–34

Miller W L 1991 Congenital adrenal hyperplasia. Endocrinol Metab Clin N Amer 20: 721–749

Nagamani M, Lingold J C, Gomez L G, Garza J R 1981 Clinical and hormonal studies in hyperthecosis of the ovaries. Fertil Steril 36: 326–332

New M I 1992 Non-classical 21-hydroxylase deficiency. In: Dunaif A, Givens J R, Haseltine F P, Merriam G R (eds) Polycystic ovary syndrome. Blackwell Scientific, Boston, M A, pp 145–161

Poretsky L, Piper B 1994 Insulin Resistance, hypersecretion of LH, and a dual defect hypothesis for the pathogenesis of polycystic ovary syndrome. Obstet Gynecol 64: 613–621

Randall V A 1994 Androgens and hair growth. Clin Endocrinol (Oxf) 40: 439–457

Regan L, Owens E J, Jacobs H S 1990 Hypersecretion of luteinizing hormone, infertility and miscarriage. Lancet 365: 1141–1144

Rodin A, Thakkar H, Taylor N, Clayton R 1994 Hyperandrogenism in Polycystic ovary syndrome: evidence of dysregulation of 11 β-hydroxysteroid dehydrogenase N Engl J Med 330: 460–465

Steinberger E, Smith K D, Rodriquez-Rigau L J 1981 Hyperandrogenism and female infertility. In: Crosignani P G, Rubin B L (eds) Endocrinology of Human infertility: New aspects. Academic Press, London, pp 327–342

Stewart P M, Shackleton C H L, Beastall G H, Edwards C R W 1990 5α-reductase activity in PCOS Lancet 335: 431–433

10

Cost-effective medical treatment of endometriosis

R. W. Stones,   E. J. Thomas

Endometriosis is a common condition in gynaecological practice but consideration of its diagnosis and management from the point of view of formal cost-effectiveness analysis has been undertaken only on a limited basis in the literature. In this review the terminology and principles of cost effectiveness and cost-utility analysis are examined. These concepts are applied to the diagnosis of endometriosis, and to its treatment in the different circumstances of pain or infertility as the main problem.

COST-EFFECTIVENESS ANALYSIS

If the outcomes of different modes of investigation or treatment of a medical condition are similar or even identical, cost becomes the predominant issue in selecting between them in a process termed cost-minimization analysis (Robinson 1993a). In practice this equality of outcome is not commonly seen, especially when side effects or complications of treatment are taken into account. In endometriosis many forms of treatment are equally effective for the relief of pain, and equally ineffective for the treatment of infertility, but there are major differences in side effects, complications and costs between different forms of therapy. Analysis of economic aspects of treatment must therefore take into account both the efficacy and drawbacks, by means of cost-effectiveness analysis. Robinson (1993b) identified the key issues in cost-effectiveness analysis as the selection of a measure or measures of effectiveness, obtaining appropriate data, the adoption of either a *risk averse strategy* where the analysis is weighted against a new or untested alternative, or *sensitivity analysis* where a model is constructed which can allow, with greater or lesser sophistication, for variation of the assumptions.

In cost-effectiveness analysis, effectiveness is measured in 'natural units', i.e. effects related to the particular disease or treatment. In endometriosis suitable measures might be relief of pain symptoms, laparoscopic evidence of resolution of lesions, or increased fertility rates. Rates of adverse response to treatment could also be included as a measure of effectiveness. A disadvantage of this approach is that value judgements have to be made between the different effectiveness measures: it may not be obvious whether the advantages of a particular treatment in terms of relief of symptoms are outweighed by the disadvantages in terms of side effects.

A further important issue is that of discounting costs and benefits over time, which depends on the perception of the investigator as to the relative benefits of good health in the near versus the distant future. For the purposes of economic analyses benefits accruing early are, by convention, considered more advantageous than longer-term benefits. Longer-term benefits have traditionally been discounted by 6% per annum, although the Department of Health and the Treasury now consider that benefits should not be discounted. The relative cost analysis will depend on the discounting assumptions used. Discounting becomes a critical issue when health interventions are proposed whose aim is to achieve a benefit many years in the future. Osteoporosis screening is a good example, as the health benefit from screening and hormone replacement therapy to prevent fractures will not accrue for 20 years or more. If a cohort of 1000 women are screened with bone densitometry it may be assumed that this will detect half the 160 women at risk of a fracture in the future. If these 80 women are given oestrogens then half the fractures could be prevented after 30 years, i.e. 40 cases. However, if this benefit is discounted at 6% then the equivalent discounted benefit is only 7 cases (Torgerson & Reid 1993).

In the context of endometriosis the question of discounting benefits is less critical but may influence strategies for prevention of disease progression: if medical therapy is not employed in early-stage endometriosis immediate costs are saved. However, there is a possibility of increased surgical costs in the future when treatment of later-stage disease becomes necessary.

COST-UTILITY ANALYSIS

Because the use of 'natural units' gives rise to difficulty in making cost comparisons between different medical conditions, methods of expressing benefit in uniform terms have been devised, for example quality-adjusted life years (QUALYs). This measure allows cost-utility comparisons to be made in standard units. Health status was analysed in terms of disability, on an eight point scale ranging from no disability through to unconsciousness, and distress; rated in four levels from no distress to severe distress (Rosser & Kind 1978). Numerical scores were then ascribed to each combination of levels of disability and distress, and this score multiplied by the number of years spent in a particular state gives the number of QUALYs.

Endometriosis becomes life threatening only in rare instances, but pain associated with endometriosis can cause disability as well as distress, rendering the sufferer unable to work or carry out household tasks. Hence alleviation of pain symptoms would score significantly in a QUALY analysis. Infertility associated with endometriosis would not usually result in disability, but generates distress. In Rosser's valuation matrix, the most severe category of distress associated with no disability, which might describe the mental state of a patient with endometriosis-associated infertility, scored 0.967. An individual with severe pain might fall into the fourth category of disability, characterized as 'choice of work or performance at work very severely limited; housewives . . . able to do light housework only but able to go out shopping'. This level of disability combined with the most severe category of distress would score 0.87. Thus in terms of QUALYs a year spent in pain with endometriosis would be valued as worth 87% of a year without symptoms, whereas a year spent in distress as a result of infertility would be worth just under 97% of a symptom-free year. This type of analysis can be used to allocate resources on the basis of maximum potential gain in QUALYs (Kind & Gudex 1993) and in the above example would favour the utilization of resources for the relief of pain in endometriosis, rather than for the treatment of infertility.

An alternative instrument for assessing health-related quality of life in a non disease-specific manner is the EuroQol© visual analogue scale, where health status is rated on a thermometer-like scale over the 0–100 range (EuroQol© Group 1990). The descriptive classification of states used in this instrument is given in Table 10.1. From these states, together with 'being dead', 16 combinations of states were derived. Scaling and validation studies were carried out by postal questionnaire, using population samples in three European countries which showed high levels of agreement in the allocation of numerical scores to each combination of health states. As examples, the median score for health states of 'no problems walking about,

Table 10.1

EuroQol descriptive classification

Mobility
        1. No problems walking about
        2. Unable to walk about without a stick, crutch or walking frame
        3. Confined to bed
Self-care
        1. No problems with self-care
        2. Unable to dress self
        3. Unable to feed self
Main activity
        1. Able to perform main activity (e.g. work, study, housework)
        2. Unable to perform main activity
Social relationships
        1. Able to pursue family and leisure activities
        2. Unable to pursue family and leisure activities
Pain
        1. No pain or discomfort
        2. Moderate pain or discomfort
        3. Extreme pain or discomfort
Mood
        1. Not anxious or depressed
        2. Anxious or depressed

no problems with self-care, able to perform main activity (e.g. work, study, housework), able to pursue family and leisure activities, moderate pain or discomfort, anxious or depressed' was 68–70, whereas for the states of 'no problems walking about, no problems with self-care, unable to perform main activity, unable to pursue family and leisure activities, extreme pain or discomfort, anxious or depressed' the median scores were between 33 and 35 in the three studies.

In a prospective economic evaluation of transcervical endometrial resection versus abdominal hysterectomy, changes in the EuroQol© score were used as a measure of health outcome (Sculpher et al 1993). Interestingly, while the mean improvement in score was significantly greater in the resection group 2 weeks postoperatively, becoming similar by 4 months, in both groups the range of change in scores included negative values, i.e. individuals who rated their health status as worse after the operation. If clinical decisions are to be based on this type of analysis it is important to know whether a change of score (especially negative) in an instrument designed to be generally applicable is indeed reflecting clinical reality. In the study cited above an interpretation more attractive to the clinician is perhaps provided in the parallel clinical paper where 'patient satisfaction' was given as an endpoint: 4 months postoperatively 84 out of 99 of the resection group compared with 89 out of 95 of the hysterectomy group reported 'satisfaction' (Dwyer et al 1993). As pressure on clinicians to justify the expense of therapeutic interventions grows, consensus on the choice and validity of outcome measures to be used is essential.

In addition to costs to the health service, costs of illness and treatment to patients and their families need to be considered. For the purposes of analysis a notional cost can be given to patients' time and included in calculations (Robinson 1993a). Illness can also directly affect the health and need for medical intervention in relatives of the affected individual. In a study of the effect of chronic pain on the children of patients, secondary costs to the health service were demonstrated: children of chronic pain sufferers had more frequent complaints of abdominal pain and used more medication than controls (Jamison & Walker 1992).

INVESTIGATION OF ENDOMETRIOSIS

When considering costs associated with the treatment of a particular medical condition it is sometimes forgotten that patients present with symptoms, and the first essential is to make a diagnosis. Overall cost effectiveness will be affected by the accuracy of diagnosis. Clinical diagnosis is a relatively cheap option but if insufficiently specific will increase the numbers inappropriately treated. Features in the history such as congestive dysmenorrhoea, and findings on examination of restricted uterine mobility or nodules in the pouch of Douglas will suggest the diagnosis of endometriosis, but large numbers of patients will not have specific symptoms or signs.

Laparoscopy has therefore become the mainstay of diagnosis. This procedure is now routinely carried out on a day-case basis, a setting in which costs are minimized by the avoidance of the need for nursing care and the infrastructure associated with an inpatient stay. On the infrequent occasions when a patient is kept in hospital unexpectedly after laparoscopy, this represents a marginal cost to the institution and does not detract from the appropriateness of the daycare concept. Alternative diagnostic methods have, however, received attention. Biochemical screening for epithelial antigens such as CA 125 has proved to be insufficiently specific, and immunoscintigraphy of lesions remains a research tool.

Early attempts were made to evaluate imaging methods as an alternative to laparoscopy for the diagnosis of endometriosis. For example, in 1985 a comparison of ultrasound with laparoscopy concluded that ultrasound was neither sensitive nor specific for the diagnosis (Friedman et al 1985). In routine practice ultrasound scanning has a place in the identification of adnexal pathology such as an endometrioma of the ovary, but is obviously not capable of distinguishing the underlying pathology. In the presence of an adnexal mass Kurjak & Kupesic (1994) have recently reported extraordinarily good sensitivity and specificity (>99%) for a scoring system combining clinical features with the biochemical marker CA 125 and transvaginal colour Doppler imaging. This system was able to identify effectively 103 cases of ovarian endometriosis in a series of 656 cases of adnexal mass. This report is unsatisfactory as it is not clear how the scoring system was arrived at. However, some of the component features are of interest. Ultrasonographic morphological features suggestive of ovarian endometrioma were thick cyst walls, regular margins and homogeneous echogenicity of cyst fluid. Using colour Doppler imaging of blood vessels, features suggestive of endometriomas were the extent of vascularization, its pericystic and hilar localization, regular separation of vessels, and a mean arterial resistance index (RI) of 0.49, standard deviation 0.11. This mean value falls between higher mean RI found in other benign ovarian tumours (with the exception of corpora lutea) and cases of pelvic inflammatory disease, and lower mean RI in malignant ovarian tumours which ranged from 0.36 to 0.38. It remains to be established whether this methodology and good results with ultrasound can be replicated in a more general setting.

A recent study from Yale University considered the cost effectiveness of magnetic resonance (MR) imaging in gynaecological diagnosis (Schwartz et al 1994). The avoidance of (expensive) surgery provided a possible means of offsetting the imaging cost of $1100 per patient in order to render it cost effective. This report contains a number of statements reflecting the North American health economic context which are unlikely to apply to European practice for the forseeable future, for example 'MR imaging is the procedure of choice in evaluation of leiomyomas . . .'. However, the authors appropriately emphasize the value of MRI for the accurate diagnosis of adenomyosis, and for distinguishing between endometriomas and other adnexal masses. In the study, 49 of a series of 69 women referred for MRI were originally recommended to have surgery to aid diagnosis or as treatment. As a result of MRI, planned surgery was either cancelled, or a less invasive procedure was performed, in 36 of the 49 women (73%). This resulted in a cost saving of $63 per patient, or $1736 per patient originally advised to have surgery.

The study also compared the findings in the 69 women undergoing MRI with a different group of 93 women undergoing diagnostic laparoscopy. Endometriosis was diagnosed in the MRI group in 8 of 69 patients (12%) and in the diagnostic laparoscopy group in 21 of 93 patients (22%). Adenomyosis was diagnosed in 12 of 69 patients (17%) of the MRI group but in none of those undergoing laparoscopy. MRI resulted in a modification of the original clinical diagnosis in 37 patients (53%), which is very similar to the effect of laparoscopy, which modified the clinical diagnosis in 55% of cases. The total cost at 1992 prices for a day-case diagnostic laparoscopy was estimated in this study at $2715, including a surgeon's fee of $1490. These costs are rather higher than those pertaining in the UK as are the MRI costs, estimated at around £550 in 1994. The analysis only included hospital charges and did not allow for costs to the patients of time off work. This might have further enhanced the apparent cost effectiveness of MRI over laparoscopy. A UK trial of this approach would be of interest.

A more down-to-earth comparison in the context of endometriosis is between the cost effectiveness of laparoscopy versus clinical diagnosis before expectant or symptomatic treatment. In the investigation of infertility laparoscopy provides additional information about tubal patency, but where the complaint is of pain it is important to consider the probability of obtaining a positive diagnosis before advising laparoscopy. Reported rates of negative laparoscopy in pelvic pain vary from 30–80% and where pathology such as adhesions or minimal endometriosis is present it is likely that this is coincidental rather than causal. The prevalence of adhesions in women with and without pain is very similar (Rapkin 1986); in endometriosis the lack of association between the stage of the disease or the site of lesions and pain symptoms has been emphasized (Fedele et al 1990) although another study from the same group reported more pelvic pain and dyspareunia, but not dysmenorrhoea, in infertility patients with stages I–II compared to stages III–IV endometriosis (Fedele et al 1992). Assuming that a careful history is taken so that other painful conditions such as irritable bowel syndrome are ruled out one could, on cost grounds, put forward a case for making a clinical diagnosis of endometriosis, supplemented by an ultrasound scan to exclude gross pathology. Medical treatment could then be instituted, and diagnostic laparoscopy reserved for those not responding.

For many patients the reassurance of a positive diagnosis is extremely important and many will decline hormonal therapy with significant side effects without the evidence of laparoscopy. The cost-benefit argument will be destroyed if expensive treatment such as a GnRH analogue is given where the diagnosis proves to be incorrect. Furthermore, it is now necessary to reconsider whether simple diagnostic laparoscopy for endometriosis is still appropriate in the light of the availability of new less invasive surgical treatments.

'ONE STOP TREATMENT'

As experience of laparoscopic methods for the treatment of endometriosis has increased, some now advocate the treatment of endometriotic lesions at the time of diagnosis, rather than as a separate procedure. This approach requires the availability of a laser laparoscope or other modalities and flexibility in the organization of operating sessions to allow treatment in an unhurried atmosphere. Until recently the efficacy of laser treatment of endometriosis associated with pain had not been established in controlled studies. Sutton and co-workers (1994) have now reported the results of a prospective randomized double-blind trial of laser laparoscopy for pelvic pain associated with endometriosis. Data on 32 women randomized to laser treatment and 31 randomized to expectant management were compared. The groups were well matched with regard to age, parity and stage of endometriosis. The improvement in pain was not significantly different between the groups at 3 months, but became significant in favour of the laser group (20 of 32 improved) at 6 months compared with 7 of 31 controls. Results in stage I endometriosis were not as good as those in stages II and III, with 6 out of 13 of the laser group reporting improvement at 6 months compared with 4 of 16 controls. The relative importance of destruction of deposits versus division of the uterosacral ligaments remains an open question as all the patients in this study underwent 'uterine nerve' transection.

There are considerable potential cost advantages in combining treatment with diagnostic laparoscopy. Lassey and Garry (1994) carried out Nd: YAG laser vaporization of endometriotic deposits at the time of diagnosis by laparoscopy, sometimes with transection of the uterosacral ligaments. They reported symptomatic improvement of dysmenorrhoea in 21 of 29 women (73%), dyspareunia in 14 of 17 women (82%) and of pelvic pain in 14 of 25 women (56%) with 19–48 month follow-up. Comparing costs, the authors contrasted the expense of laparoscopy with laser ablation (£755, including an allowance for equipment depreciation) with a diagnostic laparoscopy combined with a 6 month course of Provera (£785), Danol (£943) or Zoladex (£1327). An alternative modality is the argon beam coagulator which is cheaper and may prove to be as effective as laser laparoscopy (Daniell et al 1993).

MEDICAL TREATMENT: PAIN

In the light of recent knowledge about the efficacy of laparoscopic treatment of endometriosis the place for medical management is under scrutiny. While medical treatment is effective in relieving pain it is unlikely to eliminate disease activity and there remains a significant risk of a return of symptoms and progression of lesions once treatment is stopped. Metzger & Luciano (1989) reviewed the risks of recurrence quoted in the literature after various hormonal treatments. The risk of recurrence was not related to the choice of medication, but was greater where lower doses were used and in later stages of the disease.

Perhaps the strongest indication for medical treatment is now pain associated with minimal or mild (i.e. stages I–II) disease where laparoscopic treatment is less effective. If endometriosis recurs or progresses there is still an opportunity to carry out laparoscopic surgery and from a stage I baseline, progression to significant damage to the tubes and ovaries is less likely. Table 10.2 shows the UK National Health Service net price of a 6 month course of a range of drugs used in the therapy of endometriosis. GnRH analogues remain considerably more expensive than older alternatives. There may be scope for using lower doses of GnRH analogues, especially where pain reduction is the endpoint. Jacobson et al (1994) reported excellent symptom relief using nafarelin 100 µg bd for 6 months; half the licensed dose. 'Add-back' therapy, where a GnRH analogue is combined

Table 10.2 UK National Health Service 1994 net price of drugs used in endometriosis
Source: British National Formulary No.28

Drug Generic name	Proprietary name[a]	Dose	6 month course £ (24 weeks)
Continuous 30 µg oestrogen combined oral contraceptive pill	Examples: Ovran 30 Femodene	One daily	5.32 17.73
Dydrogesterone	Duphaston	30 mg daily[b]	71.22
Medroxyprogesterone acetate	Provera	30 mg daily	143.84
Danazol	(non-proprietary)	400 mg daily	185.14
Danazol	Danol	400 mg daily	197.88
Nafarelin (nasal spray)	Synarel	200 µg twice daily	296.80
Buserelin (nasal spray)	Suprecur	300 µg three times daily	394.90
Gestrinone	Dimetriose	2.5 mg twice weekly	438.72
Goserelin (implant)	Zoladex	3.6 mg every 4 weeks	733.62
Leuprorelin acetate (injection)	Prostap SR	3.75 mg every 4 weeks	752.24

[a] All proprietary names are registered trade marks.
[b] 20 day per month cyclical regimen.

with oestrogen or oestrogen-progestogen replacement, is effective in relieving oestrogen withdrawal symptoms (Thomas et al 1991; Gangar et al 1993) and in preventing bone loss during treatment (Leather et al 1993). This strategy has not been evaluated with regard to efficacy and long-term recurrence of endometriosis but would add only marginal cost to a 6 month course of GnRH analogue.

Mifepristone 100 mg daily reduced symptoms of pain without affecting size of lesions (Kettel et al 1994) but this agent is unlikely to be developed commercially for the treatment of endometriosis.

MEDICAL TREATMENT: INFERTILITY

Since the demonstration of a lack of effect of medical treatment of endometriosis on fertility (Thomas & Cooke 1987) numerous studies of medical and surgical treatment have attempted to show positive results. Using the methods of meta-analysis, the results of controlled trials in endometriosis-associated infertility were recently reviewed (Hughes et al 1993). The review included randomized controlled trials and cohort studies reporting pregnancies in two or more treatment arms. Thirty seven treatment comparisons were identified among 25 studies. The odds ratios for individual studies comparing ovulation suppression with no treatment ranged from 0.4 to 1.33 with 95% confidence intervals (95% CI) including unity. The overall odds ratio was 0.85 (95% CI 0.95 to 1.22). Data from six randomized controlled trials comparing ovulation suppression by means of gestrinone, a GnRH analogue or an oral contraceptive with danazol gave an overall odds ratio for pregnancy of 1.07 (95% CI 0.71 to 1.61).

These conclusively unimpressive results for medical treatment of endometriosis-associated infertility contrasted with possibly significant benefits from laparoscopic surgery which, from five studies, had an overall odds ratio for pregnancy of 2.67 (95% CI 2.08 to 3.45). The combination of danazol pretreatment with either laparoscopic surgery or laparotomy did not enhance the results compared with surgery alone. Although results from laparoscopic surgery were encouraging, significant heterogeneity was present in the studies reviewed and the meta-analysts called for larger randomized controlled trials of this treatment modality, pointing out that such trials would be feasible in a context of treatment at diagnostic laparoscopy. A recent prospective randomized study from Beverley Hills carried this approach one stage further, investigating the effect of laser laparoscopic vaporization of endometriosis at the time of gamete intrafallopian transfer (GIFT) procedures, or GIFT alone. There was no significant difference in pregnancy rates in the two groups (Surrey & Hill 1994).

In the absence of randomized trials of laparoscopic surgery for endometriosis-associated infertility, where the disease has not caused mechanical distortion of the ovaries and tubes, the appropriate management is to enhance cycle fecundity in a nonspecific manner, for example by controlled ovarian hyperstimulation and intrauterine insemination with capacitated sperm (Haney 1993). A number of studies have investigated the outcome of IVF in endometriosis compared with tubal infertility, and specifically have addressed the issue of whether medical pretreatment can improve pregnancy rates. In a retrospective analysis of IVF results in women with tubal infertility versus those with endometriosis, the pregnancy rate both per cycle and per transfer, and the implantation rate were all lower in the endometriosis group. The use of oocytes from donors without endometriosis gave similar results following embryo transfer in women with and without endometriosis. It was therefore suggested that reduced IVF success rates in endometriosis were related to the effects of endometriosis on oocyte quality (Simón et al 1994). In this study down-regulation with a GnRH analogue was employed as part of the treatment cycle. In another retrospective analysis where at least 6 weeks' pituitary down-regulation with buserelin was used before IVF, results of IVF cycles were very similar in women with tubal infertility, stages I–II and stages III–IV endometriosis (Curtis et al 1993). Thus a longer period of down-regulation appeared to enhance the results of IVF in women with endometriosis.

This approach was evaluated more formally in 84 patients with stages III–IV endometriosis (Marcus & Edwards 1994). Prior to IVF, 69 women were treated with a short protocol of GnRH analogue down-regulation followed by stimulation with human menopausal gonadotrophin and 15 received GnRH analogue pretreatment for 2–7 months before ovulation induction. The pretreatment group had 18 out of 42 (43%) pregnancies per embryo transfer compared with 17 out of 134 (13%) in those receiving the short protocol. This confirmed the advantage of reducing disease activity in endometriosis prior to ovulation induction, and lends further support to the concept of a local disturbance to oocyte development in ovarian endometriosis, rather than interference by inflammatory mediators from endometriotic deposits with fertilization and/or implantation.

In terms of cost effectiveness, accurate assessment of the mobility of the tubes and ovaries will allow selection of suitable candidates for less costly superovulation/intrauterine insemination treatment. There are no studies suggesting that GnRH analogue pretreatment confers an advantage in this context. GIFT appeared to be cost effective compared to superovulation and intrauterine insemination in endometriosis, but the reverse was true for other patient groups (Wessels et al 1992). In general IVF should be second-line treatment for endometriosis without gross tissue damage, but is the treatment of first choice for those with mechanical distortion of the adnexa. Here, GnRH analogue pretreatment has a definite role and it may be advantageous to extend the duration of down-regulation in stage III and IV endometriosis. It should be noted, however, that the allocation of particular patient groups to specific fertility treatments does depend to a considerable extent on the facilities and special skills of particular centres.

Cost-utility analysis is hard to apply in a meaningful way to infertility treatment. As discussed above, QUALY calculation shows a relatively small potential gain. Although infertility patients suffer distress, and indeed show evidence of similar psychological distress to cancer and cardiac patients (Domar et al 1993), they are not disabled. Some of the cost consequences of fertility treatment impinge on other health sectors such as neonatal intensive care for the offspring of multiple pregnancies (although neonatal intensive care itself carries a huge QUALY gain), and the theoretical hazard of ovarian malignancy in women who have had superovulation therapy may prove to be real issue in the future. The appropriate level of provision of fertility services in a publicly-funded health system is now a socio-political, rather than a strictly health economic issue.

Many purchasers in the UK health service now offer contracts for IVF/GIFT services and the basis on which services should be purchased is under discussion. A market analysis in a UK health district considered the options of purchasing via extracontractual referrals, purchasing from an existing provider either a total service or a 'transport IVF' arrangement, or establishing a new local NHS service in the area. It was noted that the costs and success rates of available facilities varied considerably, with cost per treatment cycle ranging from £498 to £2546 excluding drugs, and live delivery rates from 8.6% to 18.6% per cycle. After constructing a service specification, bids were sought with units asked to provide further information on methods and costs with their bid. GIFT was not considered to be worth purchasing as the costs were similar to IVF. It was decided to purchase 62 cycles of IVF, specifying a limit of two cycles per patient, with inclusion criteria of maternal age less than 40 and couples with nil or one child. The cost per delivery in three units submitting bids was £4085, £3253 and £3732 (Lyons 1994). Within this type of inclusive purchasing framework the inclusion of a longer period of down-regulation prior to IVF cycles for individuals with endometriosis is unlikely to be a major problem, but needs to be considered when drawing up the specification.

CONCLUSIONS

Cost-utility analysis provides a basis for decision making in the provision of health services and can also be used as an instrument for measuring treatment outcome. The application of such instruments to issues of health care provision which have a major social dimension such as infertility are limited and their role as outcome measures in clinical trials compared with traditional end points needs further study. In endometriosis presenting with pain, the traditional model of diagnostic laparoscopy followed by medical treatment now requires re-evaluation as laser laparoscopy offers the potential for cost-effective 'one stop treatment'. Where medical treatment is preferred costs range widely and, on grounds of cost, GnRH analogues remain agents of second choice. In endometriosis-associated infertility, the main role of medical therapy is ovarian down-regulation with a GnRH analogue prior to ovulation induction for IVF.

KEY POINTS FOR CLINICAL PRACTICE

- Cost-utility analysis extends cost-effectiveness analysis by using a validated scale of disease and distress expressed in a standard numerical form. This enables comparisons and value judgements to be made between different diseases and treatments.
- Ultrasonography with colour flow Doppler may have a place in distinguishing ovarian endometriomas from other adnexal pathology. Magnetic resonance imaging is the modality of choice for the diagnosis of adenomyosis. These investigations may contribute to cost effectiveness by modifying the nature and extent of surgical intervention.
- The place of medical treatment of pain associated with endometriosis is under review because of new developments in laparoscopic treatment which has now been shown to be clinically effective, especially in stage II–III endometriosis, and is also cost effective. The relative importance of laser vaporization of deposits and division of the uterosacral ligaments remains to be established.
- Before embarking on treatment the possibility should be considered that minimal endometriosis seen at laparoscopy is coincidental rather than causal in women with pelvic pain.
- The cost of a 24 week course of medical treatment for endometriosis varies between £5.32 for a continuous combined oral contraceptive preparation to £752.24 for an injectable GnRH analogue.
- Recurrence of symptoms in endometriosis is more likely where treatment has been given at a lower dose for a shorter period.
- Medical treatment of endometriosis for subfertility has been conclusively shown to be ineffective.
- Successful treatment of endometriosis-associated subfertility using IVF is enhanced by down-regulation with a GnRH analogue prior to super-ovulation. Results of IVF using donor oocytes in women with endometriosis are similar to those without endometriosis. It is likely that ovarian endometriosis has direct adverse effects on oocyte quality.

REFERENCES

Curtis P, Jackson A, Bernard A et al 1993 Pretreatment with gonadotrophin releasing hormone (GnRH) analogue prior to in vitro fertilisation for patients with endometriosis. Eur J Obstet Gynecol Reprod Biol 52: 211–216
Daniell J F, Kurtz B R, Nair S 1993 Laparoscopic treatment of endometriosis with the argon beam coagulator: Initial report. Gynaecol Endoscopy 2: 13–19
Domar A D, Zuttermeister P C, Friedman R 1993 The psychological impact of infertility: A comparison with patients with other medical conditions. J Psychosom Obstet Gynaecol 14S: 45–52

Dwyer N, Hutton J, Stirrat G M 1993 Randomised controlled trial comparing endometrial resection with abdominal hysterectomy for the surgical treatment of menorrhagia. Br J Obstet Gynaecol 100: 237–243

EuroQol Group 1990 EuroQol: a new facility for the measurement of health-related quality of life. Health Policy 16: 199–208

Fedele L, Parazzini F, Bianchi S et al 1990 Stage and localization of pelvic endometriosis and pain. Fertil Steril 53: 155–158

Fedele L, Bianchi S, Bocciolone L et al 1992 Pain symptoms associated with endometriosis. Obstet Gynecol 79: 767–769

Friedman H, Vogelzang R L, Mendelson E B et al 1985 Endometriosis detection by US with laparoscopic correlation. Radiology 157: 217–220

Gangar K F, Stones R W, Saunders D et al 1993 An alternative to hysterectomy? GnRH analogue combined with hormone replacement therapy. Br J Obstet Gynaecol 100: 360–364

Haney A F 1993 Endometriosis-associated infertility. Bailliere's Clinical Obstetrics and Gynaecology 7: 791–812

Hughes E G, Fedorkow D M, Collins J A 1993 A quantitative overview of controlled trials in endometriosis-associated infertility. Fertil Steril 59: 963–970

Jacobson J, Harris S R, Bullingham R E S 1994 Low dose intranasal nafarelin for the treatment of endometriosis. Acta Obstet Gynecol Scand 73: 144–150

Jamison R N, Walker L S 1992 Illness behavior in children of chronic pain patients. Int J Psych Med 22: 329–342

Kettel L M, Murphy A A, Morales A J et al 1994 Clinical efficacy of the antiprogesterone RU486 in the treatment of endometriosis and uterine fibroids. Hum Reprod 9: 116–120

Kind P, Gudex C 1993 The role of QUALYs in assessing priorities between health-care interventions. In: Drummond M F, Maynard A (eds) Purchasing and providing cost-effective health care. Churchill Livingstone, Edinburgh p 94

Kurjak A, Kupesic S 1994 Scoring system for prediction of ovarian endometriosis based on transvaginal color and pulsed Doppler sonography. Fertil Steril 62: 81–88

Lassey A T, Garry R 1994 Simultaneous diagnosis and treatment of early stage endometriosis. Gynaecol Endoscopy 3: ^7–99

Leather A T, Studd J W W, Watson N R et al 1993 The prevention of bone loss in young women treated with GnRH analogues with 'add-back' estrogen therapy. Obstet Gynecol 81: 104–107

Lyons C 1994 Purchasing an IVF/GIFT service for East Sussex. In: Gilman E (ed) Resource allocation and health needs: from research to policy. HMSO, London, p 95

Marcus S F, Edwards R G 1994 High rates of pregnancy after long-term down-regulation of women with severe endometriosis. Am J Obstet Gynecol 171: 812–817

Metzger D A, Luciano A A 1989 Hormonal therapy of endometriosis. Obstet Gynecol Clin N Am 16: 105–122

Rapkin A J 1986 Adhesions and pelvic pain: a retrospective study. Obstet Gynecol 68: 13–15

Robinson R 1993a Costs and cost-minimisation analysis. Br Med J 307: 726–728

Robinson R 1993b Cost-effectiveness analysis. Br Med J 307: 793–795

Rosser R, Kind P 1978 A scale of valuations of states of illness: is there a social consensus? Int J Epidemiol 7: 347–358

Schwartz L B, Panageas E, Lange R et al 1994 Female pelvis: Impact of MR imaging on treatment decisions and net cost analysis. Radiology 192: 55–60

Sculpher M J, Bryan S, Dwyer N et al 1993 An economic evaluation of transcervical endometrial resection versus abdominal hysterectomy for the treatment of menorrhagia. Br J Obstet Gynaecol 100: 244–252

Simón C, Gutiérrez A, Vidal A et al 1994 Outcome of patients with endometriosis in assisted reproduction: Results from in-vitro fertilization and oocyte donation. Hum Reprod 9: 725–729

Surrey M W, Hill D L 1994 Treatment of endometriosis by carbon dioxide laser during gamete intrafallopian transfer. J Am Coll Surg 179: 440–442

Sutton C J G, Ewen S P, Whitelaw N et al 1994 Prospective, randomized, double-blind, controlled trial of laser laparoscopy in the treatment of pelvic pain associated with minimal, mild and moderate endometriosis. Fertil Steril 62: 696–700

Thomas E J, Cooke I D 1987 Successful treatment of asymptomatic endometriosis: Does it benefit infertile women? Br Med J 294: 1117–1119

Thomas E J, Okuda K J, Thomas N M 1991 The combination of a depot gonadotrophin releasing hormone agonist and cyclical hormone replacement therapy for dysfunctional uterine bleeding. Br J Obstet Gynaecol 98: 1155–1159

Torgerson D J, Reid D M 1993 Osteoporosis prevention through screening: Will it be cost effective? Bailliere's Clinical Rheumatology 7: 603–622

Wessels P H, Cronjé H S, Oosthuizen A P et al 1992 Cost-effectiveness of gamete intrafallopian transfer in comparison with induction of ovulation with gonadotropins in the treatment of female infertility: A clinical trial. Fertil Steril 57: 163–167

11

Investigation and management of the unstable bladder

G. J. Jarvis

The concept of an unstable bladder is relatively new. In 1963, Hodgkinson and colleagues described lower urinary tract symptoms including incontinence associated with involuntary detrusor contractions in 64 neurologically normal women. The term detrusor instability was first used by Bates et al (1970). The International Continence Society (1990) defines an unstable bladder as one that is shown objectively to contract, spontaneously or on provocation, during the filling phase while the patient is attempting to inhibit micturition.

This chapter will review the aetiology and pathophysiology of the unstable bladder, together with its investigation and available methods of treatment.

BASIC CONCEPTS

The human bladder has two major functions: storage and evacuation.

The detrusor is a smooth involuntary muscle made up of a dense meshwork of fibres without any obvious stratification and the volume of the bladder at any time is the volume of urine within it. This means that the detrusor fibres must relax and stretch during the filling phase in order to accommodate the urine volume to be stored, yet must contract in order to expel that urine. Since continence is maintained because the pressure in the urethra exceeds that within the bladder, the relaxation of the detrusor during filling must be associated with a relatively unchanging intravesical pressure.

A hollow organ which allows filling and therefore an increase in volume without a coincidental increase in pressure is termed compliant. A detrusor which allows itself to be stretched without generating involuntary contractions is said to be stable and hence the definition of an unstable bladder becomes clear.

The motor activity of the detrusor is primarily under the control of the parasympathetic nervous system. This is indicated by an abundance of acetylcholinesterase activity demonstrable by histochemical staining; profuse cholinergic fibres can also be demonstrated using electron microscopy,

153

and cholinergic drugs stimulate detrusor muscle contraction. Detrusor motor neurones are found in the intermediolateral cell column in the lumbothoracic outflow of the parasympathetic nervous system and S2, 3 and 4 are the major spinal cord segments involved, perhaps S3 being the most important. Afferent fibres arising in the mucosa and surface layers of the bladder travel with the parasympathetic innovation back to the spinal cord.

The central connections between the nerve supply of the lower urinary tract and the central nervous system are complex with many discreet centres which influence micturition being described, including within the cerebral cortex, the cerebellum, the thalamus, the basal ganglia, the limbic system, the hypothalamus, and areas of the pontine reticular formation.

When the central nervous system control of the lower urinary tract is interrupted, generally by trauma, the bladder is no longer under voluntary control and unstable bladder contractions occur. In order to distinguish this situation from detrusor instability in the presence of an apparently intact nervous system, it is now convention to refer to detrusor hyper-reflexia as overactivity caused by disturbance of central nervous mechanisms; the management of these patients is outside the scope of this chapter.

The detrusor has also a sympathetic supply; pre-ganglionic sympathetic fibres with cell bodies in the thoracic and lumbar spinal segments of T^{10}–L^2 run via the superior hypogastric plexus. The sympathetic supply directly to the detrusor is relatively sparse and the exact role of the sympathetic nervous system in bladder function is unclear. It would seem that the major effect of sympathetically mediated innovation is inhibition of the motor parasympathetic ganglia within the pelvic plexus.

Since the major motor supply to the detrusor is parasympathetic, the principal neurotransmitter will be acetylcholine. For this reason, many of the drugs used in the treatment of the unstable bladder have anticholinergic activity. However, this is an oversimplification since other neurotransmitters are present which may stimulate muscle contraction and such stimulation may itself be modified by the presence of neuromodulators. The major non-cholinergic non-adrenergic transmitters which have been described include adenosine triphosphate and prostanoids, although the exact role of these

Table 11.1

Symptom	Detrusor instability	Genuine stress incontinence
Frequency	86	57
Nocturia	80	29
Urgency	92	46
Urge incontinence	88	37
Stress incontinence	26	99

substances is not known. Neuromodulators may also control the responsiveness of the detrusor to stimulatory release of acetylcholine. Those neuromodulators so far described are peptides and include vasoactive intestinal polypeptide, substance P and neuropeptide Y (Andersson 1990, Mundy 1987). It is hardly surprising, therefore, that pharmacological agents are of limited efficacy in the management of the unstable bladder.

CLINICAL FEATURES OF UNSTABLE BLADDERS

Clinicians usually associate an unstable bladder with urinary incontinence. While incontinence is a major symptom of detrusor instability, patients with unstable bladders may be continent and present with symptoms other than incontinence. Urinary incontinence itself may be caused by other pathophysiological processes which either coexist with detrusor instability or are present in the absence of an unstable bladder.

The classical symptoms of detrusor instability are frequency, nocturia, urgency, and urge incontinence. It is now recognized that stress incontinence is a symptom whereas genuine stress incontinence is a diagnosis. Patients may complain of the symptom of stress incontinence yet not have genuine stress incontinence but rather have detrusor instability. Table 11.1 shows the prevalence of these symptoms in 100 women with detrusor instability and urinary incontinence compared with 100 women with genuine stress incontinence (Jarvis 1990).

A wide range of symptoms are associated with detrusor instability and these include voiding disorders, incontinence associated with the sound of running water or handwashing, incontinence during sexual intercourse, especially at orgasm, nocturnal enuresis, and bladder pain. The symptoms complained of by 100 patients with detrusor instability are shown in Table 11.2 (Wiskind et al 1994).

The prevalence of urinary incontinence in the female population is surprisingly high, with various estimates suggesting that between 8 and 25% of all women between the ages of 15 and 65 years leak urine. This figure is surprisingly consistent for all age groups up to the age of 85 years. Women

Table 11.2

Symptom	% of patients
Urge incontinence	86
Stress incontinence	76
Frequency	53
Nocturia	48
Voiding difficulty	42
Incontinence associated with running water	30
Incontinence during coitus	14
Nocturnal enuresis	12
Bladder pain	12

delay seeking medical advice for many reasons: they hope that the symptoms will go away, embarrassment, they believe their symptoms to be normal, or are afraid of what that medical advice will be. One recent study found that only 40% of women with incontinence saw their general practitioners within the first year of symptoms, 25% delaying in excess of 5 years (Brocklehurst 1993; Jarvis 1993; O'Brien et al 1991; Norton et al 1988; Thomas et al 1980).

Various estimates are available for the percentage of women in whom detrusor instability accounts for urinary incontinence. It is difficult to quote a figure which will be consistent for all units since detrusor instability is a urodynamic rather than a clinical diagnosis and all incontinent women do not undergo a urodynamic diagnosis. However, one series estimated that 17% of incontinent women have detrusor instability as the sole cause of their incontinence and a further 17% have coexisting detrusor instability with genuine stress incontinence (Keane et al 1992). In the author's unit, 37.7% of incontinent women have detrusor instability alone whilst a further 5.2% have both detrusor instability and genuine stress incontinence (Jarvis 1994a). This suggests that between 30 and 55% of all incontinent women have an unstable bladder.

Recent studies have called into question the accuracy of such figures which may underestimate the incidence of detrusor instability. The figures quoted above arise from 'conventional urodynamic' units which diagnose bladder instability based on a filling cystometrogram performed within a urodynamic laboratory. Within the urodynamic laboratory, bladder incontinence cannot be demonstrated in 4–21% of women who claim to be incontinent (Jarvis 1994a; Keane et al 1992). The newer technique of ambulatory urodynamics in which a filling cystometrogram is performed with the patient walking about either in the hospital environment or even at home will demonstrate incontinence when none is found with the urodynamic laboratory (Davila 1994; McInerney et al 1991; Webb et al 1991). These studies have demonstrated an unstable bladder in 41 to 60% of women in whom conventional urodynamics failed to demonstrate an abnormality.

These and other studies have questioned the concept that an unstable bladder is necessarily abnormal. Robertson et al (1994) reported that up to 38% of asymptomatic volunteers have demonstrable detrusor instability on ambulatory urodynamic testing, and in the presence of detrusor instability in previously asymptomatic volunteers, only 63% experience feelings described as urgency associated with the unstable contraction, unstable contractions occurring in the absence of symptoms in 37% of such volunteers.

What does this mean in clinical practice? The single most important concept arising from the above is that an unstable bladder should only be accepted as the cause of the patient's symptoms, and therefore allowed to influence clinical judgement, if the symptoms of which the patient complains are reproduced by the urodynamic investigations.

Not all patients require a formal urodynamic assessment for the diagnosis of detrusor instability. In the absence of evidence for any other cause of symptoms, it would be acceptable in clinical practice to assume that the symptoms of urgency and urge incontinence are a result of detrusor instability. No symptoms suggestive of other urological disease should exist and no abnormalities found on urine microscopy and culture. Such patients can be treated with a clinical diagnosis of unstable bladder and referred for urodynamic investigation if they do not respond to treatment.

The analysis of symptoms shown in Tables 11.1 and 11.2, shows that in the majority of cases the clinician cannot distinguish between detrusor instability and genuine stress incontinence as the cause of the patient's symptoms. Many studies have demonstrated that, using symptoms and signs alone, between 19 and 26% of patients will be incorrectly diagnosed unless a urodynamic investigation is performed (Jarvis et al 1980; Sand et al 1988; Versi et al 1991).

From the definition of the unstable bladder the single most important investigation to be performed is a filling cystometrogram. The rationale of this investigation is that detrusor activity cannot be measured directly yet in order to diagnose an unstable bladder there must be contraction of the detrusor during the filling phase while the patient is attempting to inhibit micturition. The detrusor pressure, however, is the difference between the intravesical pressure and the intra-abdominal pressure, the bladder being an intra-abdominal structure. Both the intravesical pressure and the intra-abdominal pressure may be measured using either fluid-filled catheters or transducer-tipped catheters and the subtracted detrusor pressure obtained. In general, the bladder is filled via a urethral catheter at approximately 100 ml per minute, the patient should assume a standing position at some stage during the test, and both symptoms and incontinence should be noted. This technique is known as provocation cystometry.

Numerous other urodynamic investigations exist, including a video-cystourethrography, urethral pressure profilometry, and transvaginal ultrasonography. However, whilst these techniques may give other important information, such as the position and mobility of the bladder neck, they do not add to the confirmation or exclusion that the patient has an unstable bladder.

AETIOLOGY OF THE UNSTABLE BLADDER

In the presence of an intact central nervous system, the cause of the unstable bladder is unknown. In the majority of women with an unstable bladder, no aetiological factor can be found and the condition is assumed to be idiopathic. Several factors may be associated with an unstable bladder although such factors should not be assumed to be aetiological. In the absence of a neuropathic cause, bladder outflow obstruction and psychogenic features must be considered.

Obstructive uropathy   is undoubtedly a cause of an unstable bladder in some patients. Men with prostatic hypertrophy may have an unstable bladder which reverts to stability in most cases following relief of the obstruction (Abrams et al 1979). However, outlet obstruction is relatively unusual in women unless there has been previous bladder-neck surgery. The symptoms of hesitancy and poor stream are rarely given by women. Outlet obstruction should be considered if there is a low maximum voiding flow rate in the presence of an elevated detrusor pressure in order to produce that flow.

The commonest reason for bladder-neck surgery in women is the treatment of genuine stress incontinence. A patient can have genuine stress incontinence with a stable bladder before surgery and no longer have genuine stress incontinence following surgery yet remain incontinent because of the development of *de novo* detrusor instability. It is assumed, but not yet proven, that *de novo* detrusor instability following bladder-neck surgery is obstructive. Detrusor instability may possibly have been present preoperatively but unrecognized, or some degree of local denervation may have caused the instability. *De novo* instability may occur in 1–8% of patients following a bladder-buttress procedure, in 11% of patients after a Marshall-Marchetti procedure, in 4–18% of patients following colposuspension, in up to 20% of patients following bladder-neck long-needle suspension, and in 4–29% of patients following a bladder-sling procedure (Beck et al 1991; Jarvis 1981; Jarvis 1994b; Mainprize and Drutz 1988).

Considerable evidence suggests that an unstable bladder in women is associated with psychological dysfunction in a high percentage of patients and that such psychological dysfunction is much more likely when incontinence is caused by detrusor instability than to genuine stress incontinence. This would suggest that psychological factors are not necessarily the result of the incontinence but rather a description of the type of person who develops detrusor instability.

The evidence for the association of psychological dysfunction and detrusor instability may be summarized as below:

1. A strong emotive event in the patient's life can be the initial trigger for the urinary symptoms (Frewen 1984).

2. Patients with detrusor instability have a higher neuroticism score on formal testing than do patients with genuine stress incontinence (Hafner et al 1977; Currie & Jarvis, in press).

3. Detrusor instability shows a relationship with a hysterical personality trait (Stone & Judd 1978).

4. Patients with detrusor instability are more likely to have psychosexual problems than patients with genuine stress incontinence (Sutherst 1979).

5. Behavioural forms of therapy, for example bladder drill and hypnosis, are effective methods of treatment (see below).

6. Treatment is associated with a strong placebo effect which has been estimated as between 4 and 47% (Moore et al 1990; Meyhoff et al 1983).

These observations have an important influence upon treatment as discussed below.

THE TREATMENT OF THE UNSTABLE BLADDER

This section assumes that the condition being treated is idiopathic detrusor instability. Detrusor hyper-reflexia is beyond the scope of this chapter and outlet obstruction should be treated by the relief of that obstruction. Other causes for urgency should have been excluded by means of history, clinical examination, and examination of the urine and ideally, but not necessarily, the instability should be a urodynamic diagnosis.

The first stage in treatment should be patient explanation and reassurance. The demonstration to a patient that serious pathology has been excluded may be all that is required.

The three major options are drug therapy, behavioural modification therapy, and surgery. Two aspects are important in assessing the efficacy of different treatment modalities from the scientific literature. The first is that while the placebo response is important, the number of placebo-controlled trials are limited, and the second is that studies do not always distinguish between a reduction of symptoms and a restoration of continence.

Drug therapy has the benefit of simplicity but current drug therapy is too simplistic for the neurophysiology which exists. Most of the drugs in current practice have either an anticholinergic effect or a direct musculotropic effect, or a combination of both.

Probanthine is an anticholinergic agent and a synthetic analogue of atropine. In daily dosages which range between 45 and 145 mg, between 31 and 48% of patients will improve but not necessarily become continent; often a larger dose than this is required for a response. No strong evidence exists to show that probanthine is significantly superior to placebo, and it does have anticholinergic side effects such as dry mouth (Blaivas et al 1980; Holmes et al 1989; Thuroff et al 1991).

Flavoxate hydrochloride is generally given in a daily dosage of 600 mg although there is some evidence that 1200 mg may be more effective. Published reports suggest an improvement with treatment ranging between 0 and 58% but the anticholinergic side effects of dry mouth and blurred vision also occur (Chapple et al 1990; Gruneberger 1984; Milani et al 1988; Milani et al 1993).

Oxybutynin is currently the single most effective pharmacological agent available for the treatment of detrusor instability. This is a tertiary amine with musculotropic, anticholinergic, and local anaesthetic effects. Oxybutynin is superior to placebo and improvement rates up to 69% have been reported although continence was achieved in only 23% of patients. There is no general agreement on the best starting dose or the optimal dose which balances efficacy against side effects. The daily dosage in current use varies between 5 mg and 15 mg but up to 30 mg may be prescribed if necessary. A limited amount of evidence suggests that lower doses of oxybutynin reduce the incidence of side effects without seriously reducing efficacy (Moisey et al 1980; Moore et al 1990; Thuroff et al 1991).

Tricyclic antidepressants are interesting agents in that they are anticholinergic, sympathomimetic, and have a central sedative effect. They are particularly useful in either the anxious patient or in the patient with symptoms especially at night since they are associated with drowsiness and an improved sleep pattern. Daytime symptoms and nocturnal bedwetting have been reduced in 74% and 60% of patients respectively (Castleden et al 1981, 1986).

Synthetic vasopressin (DDAVP), given either orally or intranasally, can reduce urine production and when used at night is significantly superior to placebo in reducing episodes of nocturia and nocturnal enuresis. From the mechanism of action it clearly cannot be used for both daytime and night-time symptoms in the same patient (Hilton & Stanton 1982; Ramsden et al 1982).

Antiprostaglandins or oestrogen are no better than placebo in reducing incontinence in patients who have an unstable bladder (Wall 1990).

Behaviour modification treatment includes bladder retraining, biofeedback, hypnosis, acupuncture, and the treatment of anxiety.

Bladder retraining programmes are probably the single most effective nonsurgical treatment for the unstable bladder in women, and up to 90% of patients become continent. However, relapse is common and at the end of 3 years the success rate may have fallen to 40%. Should this occur, treatment can be reinstituted and there are no known side effects (Holmes et al 1983; Jarvis & Millar 1980).

Biofeedback is the technique by which a patient is made aware of an autonomic function using visual or auditory signals in order to demonstrate the strength of that autonomic function. The method is invasive and time-consuming; up to 40% of patients can be made continent and a further 20% improved although a recurrence of symptoms does occur (Cardozo et al 1978). Similar results may be obtained using hypnosis and acupuncture (Freeman & Baxby 1982; Philp et al 1988).

Psychological treatment for anxiety has been investigated recently as a therapeutic option in patients with an unstable bladder (Drug & Therapeutics Bulletin 1993). Using structured programmes such as counselling and formal anxiety reduction training, urinary symptoms are likely to decrease if coexisting anxiety is decreased. However, formal scientific assessment of such treatment modalities is awaited.

Surgical treatment should be reserved for those patients in whom conservative management has failed. Surgical alternatives in current practice include cystoscopy with urethral dilatation, prolonged cystodistension under regional block, transvesical phenol injections and augmentation cystoplasty.

In the absence of outlet obstruction, it is possible that cystoscopy and urethral dilatation is a placebo treatment, significantly improving between 23 and 33% of patients so-treated (Farrar et al 1976; Jarvis & Millar 1980).

Prolonged hydrostatic bladder distension produces ischaemic nerve damage when the intravesical pressure is maintained between systolic and diastolic blood pressure using a fluid column. Distension is generally performed for a 2 hour period during which time the patient is kept free of pain by either epidural or spinal anaesthesia. Up to 50% of patients may be significantly improved but the complication of bladder rupture will occur (fortunately extraperitoneal) in up to 8% of patients (Korda et al 1987; Wall 1990). In selected patients who have failed non-surgical management, bladder distension remains a useful therapy.

Transvesical phenol injection into the area of the trigone can no longer be recommended. The early results have not been replicated and a fistula can arise because of sloughing of the trigone and lower end of the ureter (Cameron-Strange & Millard 1988; Rosenbaum et al 1988).

Perhaps the most effective surgical procedure for the unstable bladder is the clam augmentation ileocystoplasty (Bramble 1982). This surgical procedure is designed to convert an unstable bladder into a hypocontractile bladder by splitting the organ in half and reconstituting the bladder using a loop of ileum on a vascular pedicle. In a recent series, 90% of patients became continent but only 75% were able to void totally spontaneously and 15% of patients had to use intermittent clean self-catheterization (Mundy & Stephenson 1985). Over and above the risks of any abdominal surgery, the other theoretical risk is that urine in chronic aposition to small bowel mucosa may ultimately induce malignancy. It is not possible to quantify this risk, since tumours take approximately 15 years to develop with ureterosigmoidostomy. Patients undergoing this procedure should be forewarned of the voiding disorder and the theoretical risk of malignancy, and annual cystoscopy is recommended.

Transvaginal electrical stimulation has been used in the treatment of the unstable bladder in Europe and to a lesser degree in North America but has not been popular in the UK. Using electrodes inserted either vaginally or anally, unstable bladder contractions may be inhibited and symptoms improved in up to 70% of patients (Bent et al 1993; Fall & Lindstrom 1994). This management has yet to be investigated by controlled trials and may not be aesthetically acceptable to all women.

CONCLUSION

Detrusor instability is a common cause of lower urinary tract symptoms, particularly incontinence in females. The aetiology is poorly understood and treatment is generally less effective than for genuine stress incontinence. Key points for clinical practice are shown in Table 11.3.

Table 11.3   Key points in clinical practice

1. Exclude pathology
2. Confirm diagnosis urodynamically, if possible
3. Explanation and reassurance
4. Drug treatment especially oxybutynin
5. Behavioural modification
6. Anxiolytic therapy
7. Prolonged cysto-distension under regional blockade
8. Clam augmentation ileocystoplasty

REFERENCES

Abrams P H, Farrar D J, Turner-Warwick R T et al 1979 The results of prostatectomy. J Urol 121: 640–642

Anderson K E 1990 Neurotransmitters in the human lower urinary tract. In: Drife J O, Hilton P, Stanton S L (eds) Micturition. Springer-Verlag, Berlin pp 29–39

Bates E P, Whiteside C G, Turner-Warwick R T 1970 Synchronous cini-pressure-flow cystourethrography with special reference to stress and urge incontinence. Br J Urol 50: 714–723

Beck R P, McCormick S, Nordstrom L 1991 25-year experience with 519 anterior colporrhaphy procedures. Obstet Gynecol 78: 1011–1018

Bent A E, Sand R K, Ostergard D R et al 1993 Transvaginal electrical stimulation in the treatment of genuine stress incontinence and detrusor instability. Int Urogynaecol J 4: 9–13

Blaivas J G, Labib K B, Michalik S J et al 1980. Cystometric response to propantheline in detrusor hyper-reflexia. J Urol 124: 259–262

Bramble F J 1982 The treatment of adult enuresis and urge incontinence by enterocystoplasty. Br J Urol 54: 593–596

Brocklehurst J C 1993 Urinary incontinence in the community. Br Med J 306: 832–834

Cameron-Strange A, Millard R J 1988 Management of refractory detrusor instability by intravesical phenol injections. Br J Urol 62: 323–325

Cardozo L D, Abrams P H, Stanton S L et al 1978 Idiopathic detrusor instability treated by biofeedback. Br J Urol 50: 21–23

Castleden C M, George C F, Renwick A C 1981 Imipramine. J Urol 125: 318–320

Castleden C M, Duffin C M, Gulati R S 1986 Double-blind study of imipramine and placebo for incontinence due to detrusor instability. Age and aging 15: 299–302

Chapple C R, Parkhouse H, Gardener C et al 1990 Double-blind placebo-controlled study of flavoxate in the treatment of idiopathic detrusor instability. Br J Urol 66: 491–494

Currie I, Jarvis G J 1994 Psychological dysfunction of incontinence. In press.

Davila G W 1994 Ambulatory urodynamics in urge incontinence evaluation. Int Urogynaecol J 5: 25–30

Drug and Therapeutics Bulletin 1993 Psychological treatment for anxiety – an alternative to drugs. 31: 73–75

Fall M, Lindstrom S 1994 Functional electrical stimulation. Int Urogynaecol J 5: 296–304

Farrar D J, Osborne J L, Stephenson T P et al 1976 A urodynamic view of bladder outlet obstruction in the female. Br J Urol 47: 815–822

Freeman R M, Baxby K 1982 Hypnotherapy for incontinence caused by detrusor instability. Br Med J 284: 1831–1834

Frewen W K 1984 The significance of the psychosomatic factor in urge incontinence. Br J Urol 56: 330–333

Gruneberger A 1984 Treatment of motor urge incontinence with clembuterol and flavoxate hydrochloride. Br J Obstet Gynaecol 91: 275–278

Hafner R J, Stanton S L, Guy J 1977 Psychiatric study of women with urgency and urge incontinence. Br J Urol 49: 211–214

Hilton P, Stanton S L 1982 The use of desmopressin in nocturnal urinary frequency in the female. Br J Urol 54: 252–255

Hodgkinson C P, Ayers M A, Drukker B H 1963 Dyssynergic detrusor dysfunction in the apparently normal female. Am J Obstet Gynecol 87: 717–730

Holmes D M, Stone A R, Barry P R et al 1983 Bladder retraining–three years on. Br J Urol 55: 660–664

Holmes D M, Montz F J, Stanton S L 1989 Oxybutynin versus propantheline in the management of detrusor instability. Br J Obstet Gynaecol 96: 607–612

International Continence Society 1990 The standardization of terminology of lower urinary tract function. Br J Obstet Gynaecol (Suppl). 6, 12

Jarvis G J 1981 Detrusor instability–a complication of surgery? Am J Obstet Gynecol 139: 219

Jarvis G J 1990 The place of urodynamic investigations. In: Jarvis G J (ed) Female Urinary Incontinence. Royal College of Obstetricians and Gynaecologists, London, pp 15–20

Jarvis G J 1993 Urinary incontinence in the community. Br Med J 306: 809–810

Jarvis G J 1994a The management of urinary incontinence. In: Jarvis G J (ed) Obstetrics and Gynaecology. Oxford University Press, Oxford, pp 260–299

Jarvis G J 1994b Surgery for genuine stress incontinence. Br J Obstet Gynaecol 101: 371–374

Jarvis G J, Millar D R 1980 Controlled trial of bladder drill for detrusor instability. Br Med J 281: 1322–1323

Jarvis G J, Hall S, Stamp S et al 1980 An assessment of urodynamic examination in incontinent women. Br J Obstet Gynaecol 87: 893–896

Keane D P, Eckford S D, Shepherd A M et al 1992 Referral patterns and diagnoses in women attending a urodynamic clinic. Br Med J 305: 808

Korda A, Kriger M, Hunter P 1987 The use of prolonged cysto-distension in the treatment of intractible urinary incontinence. Austral New Zeal J Obstet Gynaecol 27: 155–158

Mainprize T C, Drutz H P 1988 The Marshall-Marchetti-Krantz procedure. Obstet Gynaecol Surv 43: 724–729

Meyhoff H H, Gerstenberg T C, Nordling J 1983 Placebo–the drug of choice in female motor urge incontinence. Br J Urol 55: 34–37

Milani R, Scalambrino S, Carrera S et al 1988 Comparison of flavoxate in daily dosages of 600 versus 1200 mg for the treatment of urgency and urge incontinence. J Int Med Res 16: 244–248

Milani R, Scalambrino S, Millar et al 1993 Double-blind crossover comparison of flavoxate and oxybutynin. Int Urogynaecol J 4: 3–8

Moisey C U, Stephenson T P, Brendler C B 1980 The urodynamic and subjective result of treatment of detrusor instability with oxybutynin. Br J Urol 52: 472–547

Moore K H, Hay D M, Imrie A E et al 1990 Oxybutynin hydrochloride in the treatment of female idiopathic detrusor instability. Br J Urol 66: 479–485

Mundy A R 1987 Lower urinary tract structure and function. In: Mundy A R (ed) Scientific Basis of Urology. Churchill Livingstone, Edinburgh, pp 54 55

Mundy A R, Stephenson T P 1985 Clam ileocystoplasty for the treatment of refractory urge incontinence. Br J Urol 57: 641–646

McInerney P D, Vanner T F, Harris S A B et al 1991 Ambulatory urodynamics. Br J Urol 67: 272–274

Norton P A, MacDonald L D, Sedgewick P et al 1988 Distress and delay associated with urinary incontinence, frequency and urgency in women. Br Med J 297: 1187–1189

O'Brien J, Austin M, Sethi P et al 1991 Urinary incontinence. Br Med J 303: 1308–1312

Philp T, Shah P J R, Worth P H L 1988 Acupuncture in the treatment of bladder instability. Br J Urol 61: 490–493

Ramsden P D, Hindmarsh J R, Price D A et al 1982 DDAVP for adult enuresis. Br J Urol 54: 256–258

Robertson A R, Griffiths C J, Ramsden P D et al 1994 Bladder function in healthy volunteers. Br J Urol 73: 242–249

Rosenbaum T P, Shah P J, Worth P H L 1988 Transtrigonal phenol – the end of the era. Neurourol Urodynam 7: 294–295

Sand P, Hill R C, Ostergard D, 1988 Incontinent history as a predictor of detrusor instability. Obstet Gynecol 71: 257–260

Stone C B, Judd G E 1978 Psychogenic aspects of urinary incontinence in women. Clin Obstet Gynaecol 21: 807–815

Sutherst J R 1979 Sexual dysfunction and urinary incontinence. Br J Obstet Gynaecol 96: 387–388

Thomas T M, Plymat K R, Blannin J et al 1980 Prevalence of urinary incontinence. Br Med J 281: 1243–1245

Thuroff J W, Bunk E B, Ebner A et al 1991 Randomized double-blind multicentre trial of treatment of frequency, urgency and incontinence. J Urol 145: 813–817

Versi E, Cardozo I, Anand D et al 1991 Symptom analysis for the diagnosis of genuine stress incontinence. Br J Obstet Gynaecol 98: 815–819

Wall L L 1990 Urinary incontinence due to detrusor instability. Obstet Gynaecol Surv 45: 1S–47S

Webb R J, Ramsden P D, Neal D E 1991 Ambulatory monitoring and electronic measurement of urinary leakage in the diagnosis of detrusor instability and incontinence. Br J Urol 68: 148–152

Whiskind A K, Miller K F, Wall L L 1994 One hundred unstable bladders. Obstet Gynecol 83: 108–112

12

The management of postoperative voiding dysfunction

T. R. Sayer

Voiding would appear to be a simple process and is subconscious for most women. The bladder progressively fills until the tension in its walls reaches a threshold value at which time a nervous reflex, the 'micturition reflex' occurs that either causes micturition or a conscious desire to micturate. However, this simple process depends on a number of complex factors requiring careful co-ordination of bladder contraction and outlet relaxation so that bladder emptying is rapid and complete. In order to prevent or manage postoperative voiding problems the mechanics of normal voiding must first be discussed.

NORMAL VOIDING

The urinary bladder is a smooth muscle organ of two areas, the body of the bladder, and the trigone through which the ureters and urethra pass. The external muscle of the urethra is a voluntary muscle under control of the pudendal nerve. Voiding consists of bladder contraction, pelvic floor relaxation and urethral relaxation. In the female, voiding usually occurs at relatively low intravesical pressures as a result of lower outlet resistance than in the male. For some women voiding occurs at unrecordable voiding pressures. In such women a detrusor contraction may occur but pressure does not rise as the outlet resistance is so low. These women are at risk of postoperative voiding problems especially following bladder-neck surgery for stress incontinence of urine.

DEFINITION OF VOIDING DIFFICULTY

Most voiding problems in the female are often unrecognized. Standardization of terminology of such difficulties is recommended by the International Continence Society. Acute retention is where there is sudden onset of painful inability to void over 12 hours. This requires catheterization and the residual urine is greater than or equal to the normal bladder capacity. Chronic retention is more insidious and painless where catheterization gives a volume at least equal to 50% of normal bladder capacity.

165

In gynaecological surgery, acute and chronic retention may follow in two broad categories of operation. The first of these categories is where an operative procedure is performed other than for stress incontinence, and the second is postoperative retention following bladder-neck surgery. The two areas will be considered as separate issues although obviously there is overlap.

Postoperative retention

It is important to recognize over-distension as this often develops insidiously and is difficult to treat effectively. It may lead to denervation and ischaemia of the detrusor muscles and if not recognized will lead to a chronic voiding disorder. Voiding disorders are often associated with symptoms of a poor stream, poor bladder emptying, straining to void and marked hesitancy. Pain may occur with acute retention but will be absent with a chronic history of voiding disorder.

VOIDING DISORDERS IN THE GENERAL POPULATION

Bates et al (1970) first described the bladder as an unreliable witness and this is apparent in women with voiding disorders. Symptoms of voiding problems in women who have not undergone surgery are uncommon, but studies by Versi and Cardozo (1978) report an incidence of voiding disorders of 5.5% to 13% in women attending a menopausal clinic. Shepherd et al (1982) studied women with symptoms of poor voiding but found a low sensitivity of only 18% in detecting abnormal voiding using a urodynamic questionnaire. Stanton et al (1983) reported an objective incidence of voiding abnormalities of only 7%.

CAUSES OF FEMALE VOIDING DIFFICULTIES

Table 12.1 shows the most common causes of poor voiding in females. Each of these categories will be discussed further.

Some of the categories predispose patients to voiding disorders following surgery and therefore women with such factors should be carefully examined postoperatively to ensure that normal voiding has returned.

Neurological

Any patient with a pre-existing neurological problem will be at increased risk of voiding disorder after surgery. Higher lesions of the brain will often produce inappropriate voiding. Lesions of the spinal cord will have different effects depending on their level. Lesions above the level of the micturition reflex often leave the bladder hyper-reflexic with urge incontinence and poor emptying. Lesions below the reflex leave a hypotonic bladder with

Table 12.1   Causes of female voiding difficulties

Neurological	Multiple sclerosis
	Diabetes mellitus
	Cerebrovascular accidents
Urological	Urinary tract infection
	Calculus
	Urethral diverticulum
	Urethral stricture
Drugs	Anticholinergic
	Antidepressant
Constipation	
Postoperative	Immobility/Pain
	Hysterectomy
	Vaginal repair
	Bladder-neck procedure for stress incontinence
	After any surgical procedure
Psychogenic	

overflow incontinence. Radical pelvic surgery for cervical carcinoma or low colonic tumours produce variable effects on the pelvic nerve plexus and may lead to poor voiding. Diabetes mellitus predisposes the patient to a bladder neuropathy and hence to poor voiding which may be aggravated by surgery especially if a urinary tract infection occurs.

Urological

Any acute inflammatory lesion of the bladder, urethra or vagina will predispose to poor bladder emptying. Genital herpes is the most severe of these lesions. Women rarely have bladder calculi but may present with abnormal voiding particularly with an interrupted urinary stream and recurrent urinary infections. Urethral scarring as the result of recurrent urinary tract infection may lead to urethral narrowing although true urethral strictures are rare in women. Women with 'Urethral Syndrome' have frequency and urgency and on urodynamic testing will show a reduced urinary flow rate and raised voiding pressure. Such women have an inflamed urethra but in most cases no infective agent is found when the urine is cultured.

Drugs

Bladder function depends on cholinergic neurotransmission. Hence anticholinergic drugs will weaken detrusor contractility. Such drugs are atropine, probanthine, oxybutynin and tricyclic antidepressant agents. Epidural analgesia is a common cause of retention owing to the interruption of the micturition reflex arc.

Psychogenic

Urinary retention may develop in the absence of significant organic disease. Patients with psychogenic retention range from those with episodic acute retention to those who have learned to inhibit micturition (Barrett 1980). Management consists of bladder retraining with the use of clean intermittent self-catheterization as discussed later in this chapter.

Postoperative

Immobility and severe postoperative pain will predispose any patient to urinary retention. Urinary retention following vaginal repair or hysterectomy may be caused by subsequent oedema around the urethra with or without pain.

THE MANAGEMENT OF POSTOPERATIVE VOIDING DYSFUNCTION

(Non bladder-neck procedures)
Following gynaecological surgery, urinary voiding dysfunction is common. Preoperative assessment of women who may be at increased risk of problems is important and a full history will reveal women with predisposing factors such as those in Table 12.1.

The patient in postoperative retention should be catheterized with a small urethral catheter and a cause found. A catheter specimen of urine should be cultured for infection. Most women will void spontaneously after the removal of the urethral catheter 48 hours later. If the patient suffers from long-term voiding dysfunction a supra-pubic catheter should be inserted, urodynamic investigation performed and appropriate management instituted.

THE MANAGEMENT OF POSTOPERATIVE VOIDING DYSFUNCTION

(After bladder-neck surgery for stress incontinence)
Surgery for women with stress incontinence of urine is associated with a significant incidence of voiding problems postoperatively. The traditional aim of surgery is to replace the bladder neck into an intra-abdominal position, but both vaginal and supra-pubic surgery leave some women with voiding problems.

In order to understand the aetiology of voiding disorders after bladder-neck surgery the reasons for cure must be considered, but these are uncertain. Clearly, elevation of the bladder neck and an increase in urethral resistance are major factors. Coptcoat et al (1987) studied patients undergoing endoscopic bladder-neck suspension; they found an increase in outflow resistance with an increase in residual urine and concluded that although the series was small there was a trend towards bladder-neck obstruction. Stanton & Cardozo (1979) studied patients either undergoing anterior repair or colposuspension preoperatively and postoperatively. They compared the success rates for each operation and looked at the effect on voiding. The success rate for vaginal surgery of 36% was significantly less than 84% for colposuspension. However, both anterior repair and colposuspension led to significant increases in maximum voiding pressure and residual urine postoperatively. Dundas et al (1982) showed, by radiological studies of the bladder neck before and after colposuspension, that those with poor voiding postoperation had significantly reduced bladder-neck mobility. He concluded that super elevation of the bladder neck was responsible for voiding problems after colposupension.

Voiding difficulties following colposuspension have been discussed in great detail by Lose et al (1987). They found that colposuspension may introduce an element of urethral obstruction which leads to a significant proportion of immediate as well as late voiding difficulties. In their study 25% of the patients developed severe voiding difficulties in the immediate postoperative course. Of particular importance was the fact that low-pressure voiding where the detrusor pressure was less than 15 cm of water preoperatively was found to predispose significantly to immediate postoperative voiding difficulties. Another 20% of patients developed late voiding difficulties. Increased urethral resistance preoperatively was found to predispose significantly to late postoperative voiding difficulties. Lose et al (1987) emphasized that two factors are important. First that preoperative evaluation of both bladder and urethral function is vital to try to predict those women at risk of poor postoperative voiding. Second, the operative technique can result in undue overcorrection of the bladder neck, and misplacement of the sutures may create kinking or compression of the urethra during voiding.

Operative technique was investigated by Hosker et al (1991). He studied 46 premenopausal women with stress incontinence. All the women were confirmed as having pure stress incontinence by provocative cystometry and none had had any previous bladder neck surgery. At maximum cystometric capacity the women voided on a flow meter with a transurethral 7F. Gaeltec microtip transducer in the bladder recording detrusor pressure and an air-filled rectal balloon recording abdominal pressure. Bladder-neck surgery was performed on all the women. Two procedures were used: Burch colposuspension or the Aldridge fascial sling. The study compared changes in the pre and postoperative urethral pressure profile.

At the time of Burch colposuspension the sutures were inserted through the pubo-cervical fascia as classically described. However, the aim of the procedure was to support the anterior vaginal wall and bladder neck and not to cause overelevation. The assistant's fingers were placed in the vagina to push up the anterior vaginal wall such that these sutures could be tied tightly. The study aimed to avoid long-term voiding disorders and there-fore these sutures were often left bow string and to support the anterior vaginal wall only. Likewise when an Aldridge fascial sling was performed, the sling was loosely applied to the neck of the bladder in order to support and not overelevate the urethra. Bladder-neck surgery performed in this department had a cure rate of between 85% to 90%, comparable to that reported by other centres. Bladder-neck surgery had no effect on the rest-ing urethral pressures but pressure transmission rates were raised in 80% of the women following successful surgery. More importantly, as regards voiding, the results show that abdominal bladder-neck surgery had little effect on the mechanics of voiding, which is in contradiction to many pre-vious studies (Table 12.2).

Table 12.2   A comparison of pre and postoperative voiding

		preoperative		postoperative	
		Mean	(SD)	Mean	(SD)
Residual urine (ml)	Colpo.	9	(7)	30	(36)
	Sling	12	(23)	21	(31)
Max flow rate (ml/s)	Colpo.	33	(15)	28	(10)
	Sling	37	(12)	30	(13)
Urethral resistance	Colpo.	0.043	(0.07)	0.045	(0.03)
(cm $H_2O/ml^{-2}/s^{-2}$)	Sling	0.025	(0.03)	0.040	(0.04)

The results presented in Table 12.2 show that there was no significant in-crease in the residual urine following either colposuspension or a sling and no significant difference in the time between detrusor contraction and the flow commencing. The maximum flow rate was not significantly reduced and the detrusor pressure at maximum flow was not significantly altered. These findings can be summarized by the resistance ratio at maximum flow for the two principal operations performed by the supra-pubic route. Resistance ratio was not altered postoperatively in either group of patients. In summary the study showed that stress-incontinent women can be cured without creating bladder-neck obstruction.

Despite careful preoperative and operative management some patients will inevitably develop voiding difficulties. All patients undergoing blad-der-neck procedures should have the bladder drained, preferably with a supra-pubic catheter easily inserted at the time of surgery. All patients during postoperative recovery should have a CSU checked in order to detect the presence of urinary tract infection. Other general measures are to en-sure that the patient is not constipated and is mobile following her opera-tion. If the patient continues to have voiding difficulties after surgery then urodynamic investigation is easy to perform and may elucidate the prob-lems. Specific treatment involves the use of medication, surgical procedures or catheterization, principally clean intermittent self-catheterization.

Pharmacological treatment

An underactive detrusor muscle may be stimulated pharmacologically. Bethanecol chloride as a cholinergic agonist has been used for over 30 years, but its effect and efficiency has been questioned by many researchers. Wein (1980) found no effect on flow rate or residual urine and concluded there was no indication for use of this drug in women with voiding disorders. Distigmine bromide is an acetylcholinesterase inhibitor and has been reported to prevent postoperative retention but again in the long-term this medication has very little to offer in the management of voiding difficulties. Alpha adrenergic blocking agents have been considered as treatment for women with voiding disorders but as women have no evidence of innervated circular bladder-neck sphincters there is no real reason for the use of drugs such as phenoxibenzamine and prazamine. In fact their side effects are probably significantly worse than any beneficial effect that may occur.

Hormone replacement therapy may have a role in the management of postmenopausal women with voiding difficulties. Versi and Cardozo (1988) found an improvement in women treated with oestradiol implants.

Surgical management

Surgical treatment involves urethral dilatation, Otis urethrotomy or endoscopic bladder-neck incision. At all times care should be taken to avoid overdilatation and to minimize the risk of reproducing sphincter weakness or incontinence. Otis urethrotomy serves the same purpose as a simple dilatation, but certainly incisions of the urethra produce significant bleeding and require urethral catheterization until bleeding stops. These procedures only help up to 50% of women with postoperative voiding dysfunction.

Clean intermittent self-catheterisation (CISC)

If surgery does not help the patient overcome voiding disorders then the technique of clean intermittent self-catheterization should be used. Lapides et al (1972) first developed this technique from the use of sterile intermittent self-catheterization in paraplegics. Results in long-term follow-up of their patients was followed by widespread acceptance of this technique for the management of both children and adults. Murray et al (1984), in the first large group of patients treated by CISC in the UK, reported a high success rate in female retention. Patients who require this procedure should be assessed and counselled as good eyesight, manual dexterity and motivation are necessary Many different catheters can be used similar to the simple 12 French short plastic catheters which can be cleaned in warm, soapy water after use. Significant bacteriuria can be expected in up to 40% of patients but in the absence of symptoms these patients do not require antibiotic therapy. When a patient requires long-term CISC, one of the best systems available at present was developed in Birmingham, the Biscath system. This enables patients to sterilize the catheters in a simple manner by cooking them and ensure a clean catheter for catheterization.

SUMMARY

Voiding disorder is a problem which causes much distress in women, particularly following bladder-neck surgery and rapidly leads to lack of confidence in such patients. The anxiety generates further positive feedback and aggravates retention. In order to minimize this all patients should have full preoperative urodynamic assessment to assess the strength of detrusor contraction and to detect any evidence of increased outflow resistance before operation. All patients should be counselled about the possibility of long-term voiding disorders following bladder-neck surgery, especially those who may need to perform clean intermittent self-catheterization. Surgical technique is important and overcorrection causing bladder-neck obstruction at colposuspension or during a sling procedure should be avoided. Surgical techniques should aim to restore function and not to produce continence by means of obstruction.

KEY POINTS FOR CLINICAL PRACTICE

1. Before any gynaecological procedure obtain a urological history with special reference regarding predisposing factors to poor voiding.

2. Following gynaecological surgery watch for evidence of acute or chronic retention of urine and treat with catheterization promptly to prevent long-term damage.

3. All women undergoing bladder neck surgery for stress incontinence of urine require careful preoperative urodynamic diagnosis to establish their normal voiding pattern and to identify those at high risk of postoperative voiding difficulties.

4. Surgical technique is important. Do not deliberately overelevate the bladder neck. The bladder neck should be supported only and if this is done the cure rate is not decreased.

5. Postoperative problems are not treated effectively by the use of pharmacological agents.

6. Care should be taken when treating poor voiding by surgical means. Overdilatation of the urethra can lead to recurrence of stress incontinence and the inappropriate use of the Otis urethrotome can lead to urethro-vaginal fistulae.

7. Clean intermittent self-catheterization is the best way to manage women with long-term voiding difficulties after bladder-neck surgery.

REFERENCES

Barrett D M 1980 Evaluation of psychogenic urinary retention. J Urol 120: 191–192

Bates C P, Whiteside C G, Turner-Warwick R 1970 Synchronous cine/pressure/flow/ cystourethrography with special reference to stress and urge incontinence. Br J Urol 42: 714–723

Coptcoat M J, Shah P J R, Cumming J et al 1987 How does bladder function change in the early period after surgical alteration in outflow resistance?: preliminary communication. J Royal Soc Med 80: 753–754

Dundas D, Hilton P, Williams J E, Stanton S L 1982 Aetiology of voiding difficulty following colposuspension. Proceedings of the twelfth annual meeting of the International Continence Society, p 132

Hosker G L, Sayer T R, Warrell D W 1991 Does successful abdominal bladder neck surgery alter voiding? Neurourol Urodyn 10: 449–450

Lapides J, Diokno A C, Silber S J, Lowe B S 1972 Clean intermittent self-catheterisation in the treatment of urinary tract disease. J Urol 107: 458–461

Lose G, Jorgensen L, Mortensen S O et al 1987 Voiding difficulties after colposuspension. 69: 33–37

Murray K, Lewis P, Blannin J, Shepherd A 1984 Clean intermittent self-catheterisation in the management of adult lower urinary tract dysfunction. Br J Urol 56: 379–380

Shepherd A, Powell P H, Bass A J 1982 The place of urodynamic studies in the investigation and treatment of female urinary tract symptoms. J Obstet Gynaecol 3: 123–125

Stanton S L, Ozsoy C, Hilton P 1983 Voiding difficulties in the female: prevalence, clinical and urodynamic review. Obstet Gynaecol 61: 144–147

Stanton S L, Cardozo L D, 1979 Comparison of vaginal and suprapubic surgery in the correction of incontinence due to urethral sphincter incompetence. J Urol 51: 497–499

Versi E, Cardozo L D 1988 Oestrogens and lower urinary tract function. In: Studd J W W, Whitehead M I (eds) The menopause. Blackwell Scientific Publications, Oxford, pp 76–84

Wein A, Molloy T, Shofer F, Raezer D 1980 The effects of bethanechol chloride on urodynamic parameters in normal women and in women with significant residual urine volumes. J Urol 124: 397–399

13

Investigation and management of faecal incontinence

J. Hill,   E. S. Kiff

A recent survey of nearly 5000 individuals found the prevalence of faecal incontinence in the general population to be 2.3% (Nelson et al 1994). Faecal incontinence predominantly affects parous women. Therefore all obstetricians and gynaecologists will have patients with faecal incontinence. However, as there is no polite vocabulary for faecal incontinence, patients put up with disabling symptoms rather than complain. Faecal incontinence secondary to birth trauma may result from direct injury to the anal sphincter musculature, injury to the nerve supply of the anal canal and pelvic floor muscles or injuries to both muscle and nerve. The resulting incontinence may present at any time from immediately after delivery to many years later. An understanding of faecal incontinence aids the complete assessment of any condition associated with pelvic floor dysfunction such as uterine prolapse and urinary incontinence.

PHYSIOLOGY

Continence implies that the contents of the bowel are contained within it and therefore anal pressure must at all times be greater than rectal pressure. Anal pressure is produced by complementary activity of the internal anal and external anal sphincter muscles. Rectal pressure increases as it distends and also with increased intra-abdominal pressure which may be sudden. There are therefore systems to detect these changes and to compensate for them in order to maintain continence. Failure of any part of these systems may lead to faecal incontinence.

The anal sphincter complex comprises the internal anal sphincter muscle and the voluntary sphincter muscles. The internal anal sphincter is under autonomic control, usually in a state of continuous although fluctuating contraction and is responsible for 75% of the resting tone in the anal canal (Frenkner & Von Euler 1975). Its action prevents leakage of rectal contents between bowel actions. The voluntary sphincter comprises the external anal sphincter and puborectalis muscles. The external anal sphincter is a cylinder of striated muscle which surrounds the internal anal sphincter and is innervated by the pudendal nerves (S2, S3 and S4) (Fig. 13.1). The

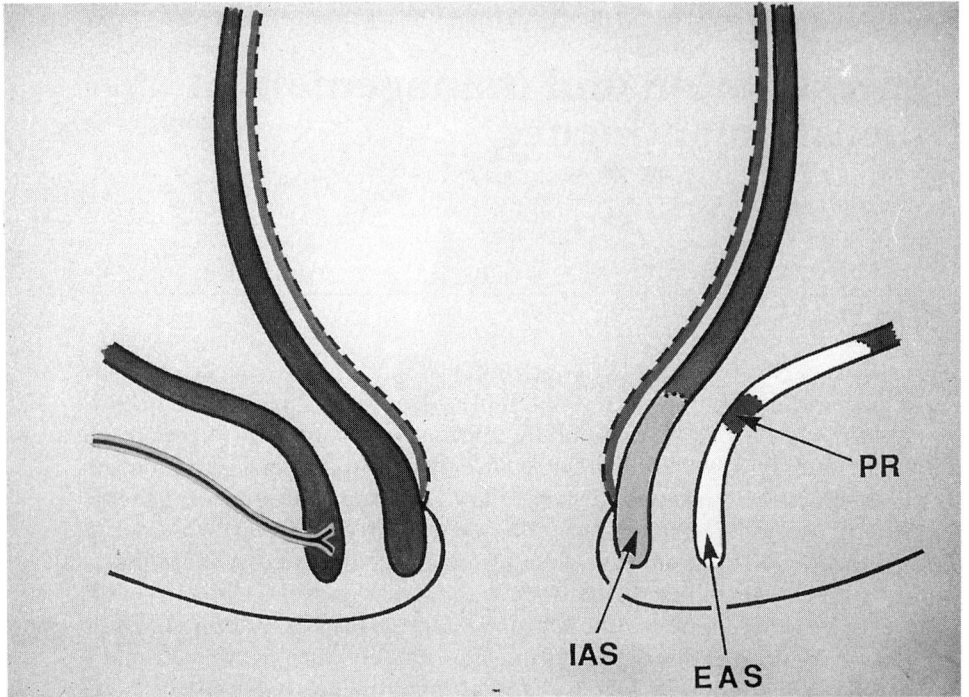

Fig. 13.1   Schematic diagram of the anal sphincter complex and pudendal nerve.

external sphincter muscle is able to double the anal canal pressure (voluntary squeeze pressure) and is used to defer defaecation. The resting pressure of the anal canal and the voluntary squeeze pressure decrease with age and both are lower in women compared with men (McHugh & Diamant 1987; Jameson et al 1994). As a group, incontinent patients have lower resting pressures and voluntary squeeze pressures in the anal canal than continent patients, however, there is considerable overlap and continence relies on a balance of all the physiological factors mentioned.

Continence is also maintained by the puborectalis muscle and the other pelvic floor muscles. The puborectalis is innervated by pelvic branches of the sacral plexus (S3 and S4), is attached to the back of the symphysis pubis and runs around the anorectal junction. In normal women the puborectalis maintains an angle of 60 to 130° between the anal canal and lower rectum (Shorvon et al 1989). Although the precise mechanism of action is unclear, puborectalis acts with the other pelvic floor muscles to raise the pelvic floor, on average by 1 cm, during squeezing when patients are deferring defaecation. During defaecation, the pelvic floor descends, on average by 2 cm, and the anal canal widens and shortens (Shorvon et al 1989).

Continence is further aided by a spinal reflex that results in contraction of the voluntary sphincter muscles during sudden increases in intra-abdominal pressure. The integrity of this spinal reflex can be established during digital rectal examination by asking the patient to cough (the cough reflex). Normal sensation in the anorectum is also important. Sensory receptors in the pelvic floor detect the presence of rectal distension. The sensory receptors in the anal canal are capable of discriminating between flatus, liquid and solid stool. The anal sphincter muscles are thought to relax momentarily in the process of sampling, when a small sample of rectal contents passes into the anal canal.

FACTORS PREDISPOSING TO FAECAL INCONTINENCE

These are listed in Table 13.1. The striated muscles are under voluntary control and their normal function is dependent on intact higher centres. Thus, neurological causes of incontinence include disturbances of central nervous system function such as dementia, stroke, spinal cord lesions including myelomeningocoele, neoplasms and trauma.

Conditions such as inflammatory bowel disease, diverticular disease, radiation enteritis and laxative abuse all cause loose stools, stress the continence mechanism and predispose to faecal incontinence.

Rectal disease may lead to loss of rectal compliance and thus loss of its reservoir function. This may be seen in association with chronic proctitis, after pelvic irradiation and following rectal surgery.

Faecal impaction leading to overflow incontinence has many causes including dementia, institutionalization, postoperative pain, opiate and anti-diarrhoeal usage. The patient leaks liquid stool around the site of the impacted ball of solid stool.

Table 13.1 Factors predisposing to faecal incontinence

Neurological	Dementia, cerebrovascular accident
	Spinal cord lesions
	Neurogenic faecal incontinence
Trauma	Obstetric
	Anorectal surgery
	Accidental
Rectal disease	Prolapse
	Loss reservoir function
	Carcinoma
	Faecal impaction
Conditions causing loose stools	Diverticular disease
	Infectious enteritis
	Inflammatory bowel disease
	Irritable bowel syndrome
	Radiation enteritis
	Laxative abuse

About half of the patients with a full thickness rectal prolapse are incontinent of faeces. The incontinence results from associated pelvic floor weakness, chronic stretching of the anal sphincter and mucous discharge from the prolapsed mucosa. Rectal prolapse can occur in young people and may be missed. Patients with prolapse of the rectal mucosa alone may also present with incontinence. It is usually mild and consists of leakage of small volumes of liquid stool and mucus at the site of the prolapsing mucosa.

An important neurological disorder causing faecal incontinence is idiopathic, also called neurogenic, faecal incontinence. This is characterized by peripheral neuropathy of the pudendal nerve and denervation of the pelvic floor, with subsequent weakness of the striated muscles of the pelvic floor and external anal sphincter. Pudendal neuropathy is also associated with urge incontinence of urine. A subgroup of these patients also have weakness of the autonomically innervated internal anal sphincter (Sun et al 1989). The reasons for this are not yet precisely determined, but in this group of patients, incontinence tends to be more severe.

Any physical injury to the anal sphincter complex may result in impaired function, however, minor injuries do not usually cause severe incontinence. Trauma to the anal sphincter occurs most commonly during vaginal delivery and colorectal surgery.

Effect of vaginal delivery on the pelvic floor and anal sphincter

A recent study found that third degree perineal tears, resulting in overt anal sphincter damage occurred in 0.5% of vaginal deliveries (Sultan et al 1993a). This study identified forceps delivery as a major risk factor for third degree tears. Anorectal ultrasound performed before and after vaginal delivery has identified a much higher rate of occult injury to the anal sphincter. Sultan et al (1993b) found that 35% of primiparous women and 44% of multiparous women had a sphincter defect after vaginal delivery. As there was only a 4% increase in sphincter damage after delivery in the multiparous group, most of whom had only had one vaginal delivery, the risk of sphincter damage seemed to be greatest during the first delivery. Perhaps surprisingly, the internal sphincter was injured more frequently than the external sphincter and sometimes even when the perineum remained intact. The mechanism for this injury is unknown, but may be related to shearing forces produced by the descent of the baby's head. External sphincter damage occurred only in association with a perineal tear or episiotomy. Injury to both the internal and external sphincter involved the entire length of the sphincter in the majority of cases.

In their study, Sultan et al (1993b) also found that structural damage to the sphincters persisted 6 months later suggesting that this damage is permanent. Perhaps most importantly they found a definite relationship between sphincter defects, anal pressure, faecal urgency and faecal incontinence. Six weeks after delivery, 28 of 39 women with a sphincter defect had faecal urgency or faecal incontinence, compared with 1 of 78 women who had no sphincter defect.

Episiotomy does not protect the mother from suffering a sphincter injury, however, anal sphincter injury is significantly more common after midline episiotomy than after mediolateral episiotomy (Coats et al 1980). Studies have suggested an upper limit for overall rates of episiotomy in spontaneous vaginal deliveries of 20–30% (Henriksen et al 1992; Argentine Episiotomy Trial 1993). Reducing the overall rates substantially below this level may be associated with an increased risk of anal sphincter injury (Henriksen et al 1994). Instrumentally-assisted delivery is also associated with a significantly greater risk of anal sphincter injury. This risk may be reduced if vacuum extraction is used. Johanson et al (1993), in a randomized study, found third-degree tears occurred in 5% of vacuum extractions and in 8% of forceps extractions. There were significantly fewer women with anal sphincter damage or upper vaginal extensions in the vacuum extractor group.

Damage to the innervation of the pelvic floor also occurs during childbirth as a result of stretching at the time of perineal descent. Snooks et al (1984) found evidence of damage to the pudendal nerve in 42% of women 2 to 3 days after vaginal delivery, but in none of the women who were delivered by caesarian section. Pudendal nerve damage was more common and more severe in multiparae delivered vaginally. Although the pudendal nerve conduction studies showed recovery by 2 months after delivery, they also found evidence of re-innervation of the external anal sphincter. Re-innervation is associated with an external sphincter weakness and implies neuronal loss. Allen et al (1990) also found partial denervation (with consequent re-innervation) in the pelvic floor muscles after vaginal delivery. Both studies found that nerve damage was greater when the second stage of labour was prolonged. There is evidence that the neuropathy persists and may become more marked 5 years after vaginal delivery (Snooks et al 1990). To make matters worse, damage to the innervation of the external anal sphincter often co-exists with direct injury to the muscle (Snooks et al 1985). The neuropathy that occurs during vaginal delivery is also thought to occur where there is repetitive chronic perineal descent, such as straining at stool because of chronic constipation or the descending perineum syndrome. Longitudinal studies have demonstrated that pudendal neuropathy increases in patients with idiopathic faecal incontinence with a parallel fall in the voluntary squeeze pressures in the anal canal (Hill et al 1994a).

Effect of colorectal surgery on the anal sphincters and pelvic floor

The ability to assess anorectal function based on a history and physical examination should be possessed by anyone intending to operate on the anorectum. This ability also helps in the complete assessment of any condition associated with pelvic floor dysfunction such as uterine prolapse and urinary incontinence. Several 'minor' colorectal procedures can affect anorectal function. Anal dilatation is performed by digitally stretching the anal sphincter under general anaesthetic for the treatment of anal fissure and haemorrhoids. This procedure tears fibres of the internal anal sphincter muscle and results in permanent reduction of the resting pressure in the anal canal. As it is now recognized to result in an uncontrolled injury to the anal sphincter, most colorectal surgeons now perform an alternative procedure. Lateral sphincterotomy also results in a permanent reduction of the resting pressures in the anal canal, but it is a controlled division of the lower part only of the internal anal sphincter. In a large series of internal anal sphincterotomies reported by Khubchandani & Reed (1989), 5.3% reported accidental bowel movements and 4% regularly wore absorbent pads.

A variety of surgical techniques are used to treat patients with fistula in ano, the commonest treatment being laying open of the fistula track. Fistulas involving the lower half of the anal canal can usually be treated without risk of incontinence. This is not the case for higher fistulas, where other strategies are used such as: staged division of the fistula track, the use of setons (suture material inserted into the fistula track) or the use of a defunctioning colostomy.

Many patients experience minor degrees of faecal incontinence after anterior resection of the rectum and after ileoanal pouch operations. This usually improves during the first year after operation.

CLINICAL ASSESSMENT

Clinical evaluation will identify most causes of faecal incontinence. Important details in the history are shown in Table 13.2. The severity of incontinence is determined by the frequency of incontinent episodes (both day and night), the requirement and number of incontinence pads used and the restriction of normal activities. Severity is also graded according to loss of control for flatus, liquid or solid stool. The stool consistency is particularly important, as loose stools may expose a relatively minor weakness of the anal sphincter. Leakage of small volumes of stool between defaecatory episodes indicates weakness of the internal anal sphincter muscle. The inability to defer defaecation with incontinence en route to the lavatory indicates weakness of the voluntary sphincter complex (Hill et al 1994b). Co-existing urge incontinence of urine is also associated with voluntary sphincter weakness. The presence of any neurological symptoms should be ascertained. Details of previous surgery to the anal canal, gastrointestinal tract, drug therapy and associated medical diseases are recorded. The relevant obstetrical history includes the number of vaginal deliveries, the use of forceps and episiotomy, difficult or prolonged labour and the

Table 13.2   Relevant history in patients with faecal incontinence

Length of history
Stool frequency
Stool consistency
Urgency
Incontinent en route
Severity: minor
        working
        out with difficulty
        confined
Events provoking incontinence:
        exercise
        coughing
        intercourse
Leakage: flatus
        liquid
        solid
Number of pads per 24 hours
Urinary incontinence
Obsteric history
Operations: genitourinary
        colonic
        anorectal

occurrence of perineal tears. A general examination should then be performed including a neurological examination. Inspection of the perineum may reveal the presence of faecal soiling, perianal excoriation, fistulae, scars from previous perianal sepsis, episiotomies or tears. A cutaneous anal reflex elicited by stroking or scratching the skin near the anus results in contraction of the external sphincter and indicates the integrity of the third and fourth sacral segments. The patient should then be asked to strain, the observer looking for perineal descent and prolapse. Gaping of the anus on traction of the anal verge indicates weakness of the internal anal sphincter. Digital examination may detect the presence of faecal impaction (a hard ball of faeces filling the rectum) or a low rectal carcinoma. With experience an accurate assessment of internal anal sphincter function (indicated by the resting tone) and the voluntary sphincter muscle function (by asking the patient to squeeze the examining finger) can be made. The anorectal angle and the presence of a cough reflex should be determined (Table 13.3).

Typically in a woman with neurogenic incontinence one would see gaping of the anus on traction, perineal descent on straining, the anal canal would be short in length and there would be a poor anorectal angle with little or no movement on voluntary contraction. This would imply weakness of both internal anal sphincter muscle as well as the voluntary muscle complex. The latter results in the perineal descent, shortening of the anal canal and loss of the anorectal angle. There will always be symptoms with these findings but the patient will often conceal them unless asked directly.

Table 13.3   Perianal examination of patients with faecal incontinence

Inspection	Scars/fistulae
	Excoriation
	Anal reflex
	Perineal descent
	Mucosal prolapse
	Gaping of the anal canal
Digital examination	Faecal impaction
	Carcinoma
	Resting tone
	Voluntary contraction
	Anorectal angle
	Cough reflex

INVESTIGATIONS

All patients should have a proctoscopy and sigmoidoscopy which can be performed at the first outpatient visit. Proctoscopy is particularly valuable when mucosal prolapse is suspected. The colon must then be examined by either colonoscopy or barium enema examination in order to exclude more sinister causes of diarrhoea.

Further information is provided by anorectal physiological studies and by radiological examination. These tests are valuable in that they are objective, reliable, accurate and reproducible (Kiff 1983; Rogers et al 1989). They usually confirm the clinical impression, may be repeated to assess the efficacy of therapy and may be of value medico-legally.

Manometry of the anal canal is performed using a variety of techniques including water perfused catheters, air and water-filled balloons and solid-state microtransducer pressure catheters. The resting tone in the anal canal (normal range 45–97 cm H_2O), and voluntary contraction pressures (normal range 76–258 cm H_2O) are measured at 1 cm intervals. The anal canal length can thus be determined and is normally 3 to 4 cm.

The technique of electromyography is performed by inserting fine needles into the voluntary sphincter muscles. This is done circumferentially with concentric EMG needles to identify any trauma induced gaps in the muscle ring or using single fibre EMG to measure fibre density in these muscles. Fibre density is increased in pudendal neuropathy and indicates re-innervation.

Pudendal nerve terminal motor latency is measured using a rubber finger stall with two metal stimulating electrodes at its tip and two metal surface electrodes for recording mounted at its base. The finger stall is inserted into the anal canal and the pudendal nerve stimulated as it passes close to the ischial spine. The time taken for the impulse to travel along the terminal portion of the pudendal nerve and contract the external sphincter muscle is recorded bilaterally (Kiff & Swash 1984). The pudendal nerve terminal motor latency is typically increased in neurogenic (idiopathic) faecal incontinence. A prolonged pudendal nerve terminal motor latency indicates significant damage to the nerve supply of the external anal sphincter muscle.

A variety of methods have been described to measure sensation in the anal canal and rectum. They have increased our understanding of physiological functioning of the anal canal. Loss of anal sensation is associated with the development of incontinence (Miller et al 1989). Anal canal sensation is also a function of the pudendal nerves and therefore loss of sensation also implies a pudendal neuropathy.

Defaecating proctography and cinedefaecography are performed by inserting barium paste or a barium-filled condom into the rectum. The patient is asked to contract the anal sphincter then to evacuate the barium. The former technique records static images and in defaecography images are recorded on videotape. From the images, the anorectal angle, perineal descent and anal canal length can be measured. In addition the technique detects the presence of a rectocoele, complete or partial rectal prolapse, and assesses the completeness of rectal emptying.

Anorectal ultrasound imaging has been developed during the last 5 years and is replacing concentric needle electromyography as a technique to

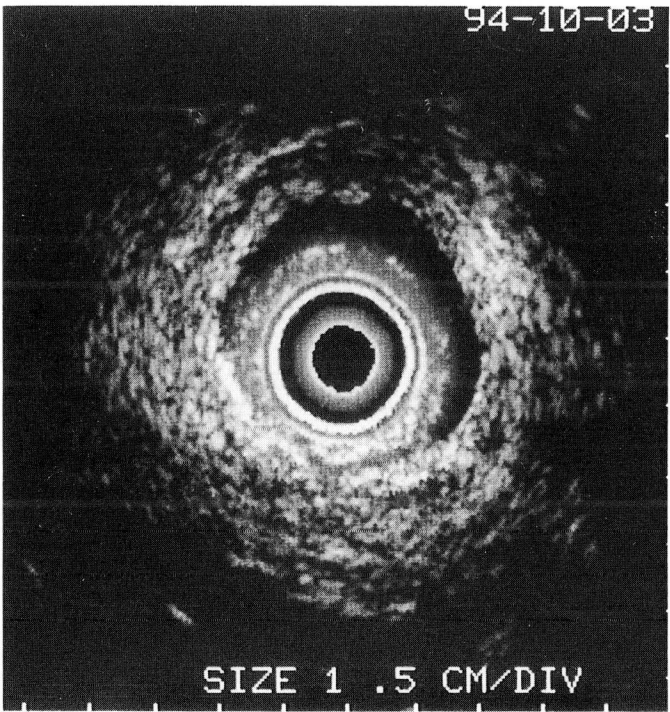

Fig. 13.2 Anal canal ultrasound demonstrating a defect in the internal anal sphincter muscle indicated by a loss of the hypoechoic ring.

identify anatomical defects in the anal sphincter musculature. A rotating rectal probe (focal range 2–5 cm) covered with a plastic cone is inserted into the anal canal. Ultrasound provides an accurate anatomical assessment of the anal canal musculature, including puborectalis. Defects in the muscle are identified by breaks in the normal texture of the muscle rings (Figs 13.2 and 13.3).

TREATMENT

Conservative therapy

Medical treatment has an important role in the management of faecal incontinence. The commonest clinical presentation encountered is the middle aged or elderly female patient who has a minor or moderate weakness of the voluntary sphincter that is exposed by the development of loose stools. The patient is unable to defer defaecation, is incontinent en route to the toilet and has to alter her daily routine to avoid accidents. Antidiarrhoeal therapy alone may be sufficient to restore continence. Loperamide and codeine phosphate are used initially. The former drug may have

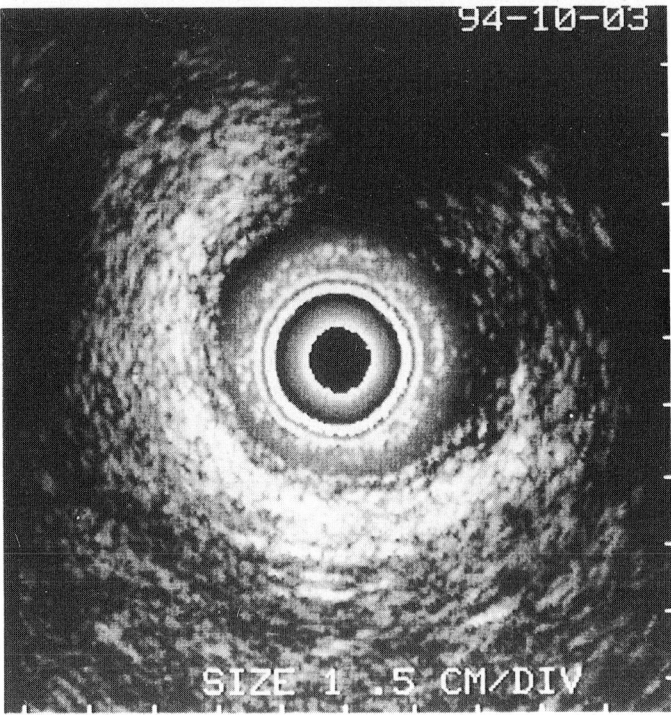

Fig. 13.3 Anal canal ultrasound demonstrating a defect in the external anal sphincter indicated by a break in the normal hypoechoic outer ring.

a specific action on the anal sphincter to increase resting pressure (Read et al 1982). Any existing medical condition that causes loose stools, such as inflammatory bowel disease, should be treated. The addition of a bulking agent and a high-fibre diet usually produces soft formed stools although in some patients fibre results in overtly loose stools. All other treatment of faecal incontinence will be maximized by attaining a solid-formed stool and this factor should not be forgotten when comparing the efficacy of different treatments.

Faecal impaction is treated with enemas and manual evacuation, a general anaesthetic frequently being necessary in order to do this. Impaction is liable to recur unless regular laxatives and suppositories or enemas are administered.

Biofeedback training has been used widely to treat faecal incontinence. Although the techniques vary slightly, the principle is that patients are taught to recognize rectal distension and then to contract their voluntary sphincters during the phase of reflex reduction in internal sphincter activity. The rectum is distended with increasing volumes of air in a rectal balloon. The EMG trace and the pressure generated by the external anal sphincter muscle are recorded and displayed on a screen. The patient is able to watch the images on the screen as the sphincter is contracted and learn how to maximize their muscular effort. Reports have suggested that two-thirds of incontinent patients are significantly improved using biofeedback techniques (MacLeod 1987). How this is achieved is not entirely clear as there is no demonstrable increase in sphincter pressures after biofeedback training. It is least beneficial in patients with very poor sphincter function. Biofeedback is time consuming and requires a dedicated patient and therapist.

Surgical management

Prolapse

Prolapse of the rectal mucosa alone is treated with rubber band ligation, injection with sclerosants or excision. More than 100 operations have been described to treat full-thickness rectal prolapse. The commonest procedure performed from the perineal approach in the United Kingdom is Delormes operation. In this, the mucosa of the prolapsed bowel is excised and the muscularis propria of the prolapsed bowel is plicated. This procedure can be performed under regional anaesthesia. The abdominal approach also carries a low morbidity and mortality. The rectum is mobilized and fixed to the sacrum by sutures, a mesh or a sling. Correction of the prolapse improves or resolves incontinence in most patients although some patients do experience difficulty in defaecation postoperatively. Rectopexy can be safely performed even in very elderly patients and greatly facilitates the nursing care of institutionalized patients with this condition (Mann & Hoffman 1988).

Sphincter repair

Accurate primary repair of obstetric injury to the anal sphincter is a technically difficult procedure indicated by the reported faecal incontinence rates of 30 to 50% in follow-up studies (Nielsen et al 1992; Sorensen et al 1988; Haadem et al 1987). A recent study using anal ultrasound in the follow-up of primarily sutured sphincteric ruptures demonstrated a defect in the external sphincter in 13 of 24 patients. Six of the 13 were incontinent, in comparison with one patient in the 10 patients with a normal ultrasound (Nielsen et al 1992). Primary repair usually fails because of a combination of unrecognized injury, sepsis or faulty technique. These studies perhaps suggest that a more senior surgeon, preferably one who is familiar with the anal sphincter, should perform the primary sphincter repair. In the event of a particularly extensive perineal wound, a diverting colostomy may be necessary with a delayed sphincter repair performed three months later. This is more often required for sphincter injuries occuring as a result of road traffic accidents.

Nielsen et al (1992) suggest that women who have a demonstrable defect in the external sphincter be informed of the risk of further perianal trauma and possibly be offered a caesarian section. Patients who have had ileoanal pouch procedures tend to have lower anal canal sphincter pressures and a liquid/semi-solid stool and are thus at risk of faecal incontinence. It has been suggested that this group of patients should also be delivered by caesarian section for any subsequent delivery. As yet, there is no hard data to support these suggestions and each case must be evaluated individually. It seems logical, however, to avoid vaginal delivery where an injured sphincter has already been repaired.

Most sphincter repairs are performed as secondary procedures, months or years after primary repair. The principles of sphincter repair are to mobilize the external sphincter widely and to divide and preserve the scar tissue (this holds sutures better than the sphincter muscle itself). The cut ends are then overlapped and sutured in place. Superficial infection is common but only rarely does infection compromise the repair. Results of repair are generally good, with about 80% of patients regaining continence of solid stool. Poorer results are reported for those patients with co-existent pelvic floor neuropathy indicated by impaired pudendal nerve function (Laurberg et al 1988). As for primary repair, a defunctioning colostomy is rarely indicated for obstetric injuries, but it is mandatory when repairing a sphincter following fistula surgery where the extent of muscle loss is greater.

Postanal repair

The technique of postanal repair was was first described by Parks in 1959 (Parks 1975). It was designed to treat patients with a weak but intact pelvic floor and anal sphincter, and therefore is usually performed on patients with neurogenic (idiopathic) faecal incontinence. The operation is performed by opening the intersphincteric space posteriorly (between internal and external anal sphincter muscles) to gain access to the levator muscles of the pelvic floor. The levator ani, puborectalis and external anal sphincter muscles are plicated posteriorly using nonabsorbable sutures. A recently reported long-term study of postanal repair has demonstrated that two-thirds of patients maintained markedly improved continence at 5 years although only 26% achieved restoration of normal continence (Setti Carraro et al 1994). As for sphincter repair, impaired pudendal nerve function is a predictor of poor outcome (Laurberg et al 1990). No other surgical procedure has proved effective for this group of patients, thus postanal repair has an important role in the management of idiopathic faecal incontinence.

For patients who fail after treatments listed above, a few remedial options remain. An implantable artificial anal sphincter which encircles the anal canal has been designed. A subcutaneous pump is used to fill an inflatable cuff that occludes the anal canal (Christiansen & Lorentzen 1989). Very few of these devices have been inserted, and more optimism currently exists for the technique of encircling the anal canal with the gracilis muscle (Williams et al 1991). The nonstimulated gracilis muscle neosphincter improves continence in the majority of patients (Faucheron et al 1994). The addition of chronic electrostimulation improves the function of the transposed gracilis muscle with correspondingly better results, restoring continence in 60–100% of patients (Williams et al 1991; Seccia et al 1994).

A disposable anal continence plug has also been developed. Early results were encouraging, but the plugs are not currently commercially available (Mortensen & Humphreys 1991). Techniques of anal encirclement such as the Thiersch wire are now rarely performed. If all else fails, a colostomy or ileostomy should be considered as they may considerably improve the quality of life in a patient with intractable incontinence.

KEY POINTS FOR CLINICAL PRACTICE

1. Faecal incontinence predominantly affects parous women. All obstetricians and gynaecologists will have patients who suffer from faecal incontinence.

2. Many patients will not confess to faecal incontinence unless specifically asked.

3. An appropriate history and examination leads to an accurate assessment of the cause of faecal incontinence in the majority of cases.

4. A high rate of occult injury occurs to the internal and external anal sphincter after spontaneous vaginal delivery. The risk is greatest during the first delivery.

5. Episiotomy does not protect the mother from sphincter injury; high and low rates of episiotomy are associated with a greater risk of sphincter injury. The optimum episiotomy rate seems to be 20 to 30%.

6. Damage to the innervation of the pelvic floor also occurs during childbirth. The risk is greater when the second stage of labour is prolonged. The neuropathy may persist and worsen with time.

7. Anorectal physiology studies are accurate and repeatable. Pudendal neuropathy is a bad prognostic indicator for surgical outcome after sphincter repair and postanal repair.

8. Conservative treatment with antidiarrhoeal therapy is an effective treatment for many patients with loose stools and faecal incontinence.

9. Primary sphincter repair is technically difficult and should ideally be performed by a surgeon familiar with the anal canal musculature.

10. Results of secondary sphincter repair are generally good with about 80% of patients regaining continence of solid stool.

REFERENCES

Argentine Episiotomy Trial Collaborative Group 1993 Routine vs selective episiotomy: a randomised controlled trial. Lancet 342: 1517–151
Allen R E, Hosker G L, Smith A R B et al 1990 Pelvic floor damage and childbirth: a neurophysiological study. Br J Obstet Gynaecol 97: 770–779
Coats P M, Chan K K, Wilkins M et al 1980 A comparison between midline and mediolateral episiotomies. Br J Obstet Gynaecol 87: 408–412
Christiansen J, Lorentzen M 1989 Implantation of artificial sphincter for anal incontinence. Dis Colon Rectum 32: 432–436
Faucheron J L, Hannoun L, Thome C et al 1994 Is fecal incontinence improved by nonstimulated gracilis muscle transposition? Dis Colon Rectum 37: 979–983
Frenckner B, Von Euler C 1975 Influence of pudendal block on the function of the anal sphincters. Gut 16: 482–489
Haadem K, Dahlstrom A, Ling L 1987 Anal sphincter function after delivery rupture. Obstet Gynecol 70: 53–56
Henriksen T B, Bek K M, Hedegaard M, Secher N J 1992 Episiotomy and perineal lesions in spontaneous vaginal deliveries. Br J Obstet Gynecol 99: 950–954
Henriksen T B, Bek K M, Hedegaard M, Secher N J 1994 Methods and consequences of changes in use of episiotomy. 309: 1255–1258
Hill J, Corson R J, Brandon H et al 1994a History and examination in the assessment of patients with idiopathic fecal incontinence. Dis Colon Rectum 37: 473–477
Hill J, Mumtaz H, Kiff E S 1994b Idiopathic faecal incontinence–pudendal neuropathy progresses with time. Br J Surg 81: 1492–1494
Jameson J S, Chia Y W, Kamm M A et al 1994 Effect of age sex and parity on anorectal function. Br J Surg 81: 1689–1692
Johanson R B, Rice C, Doyle M et al 1993 A randomised prospective study comparing the new vacuum extractor policy with forceps delivery. Br J Obstet Gynaecol 100: 524–530
Kiff E S 1983 The clinical use of anorectal physiology studies. Ann R Coll Surg Engl 1 (Suppl) : 27–29
Kiff E S, Swash M 1984 Slowed conduction in the pudendal nerve in idiopathic (neurogenic) faecal incontinence. Br J Surg 71: 614–616
Khubchandani I T, Reed J F 1989 Sequelae of internal sphincterotomy for chronic fissure in ano. Br J Surg 76: 431–434
Laurberg S, Swash M, Henry M M 1988 Delayed external sphincter repair for obstetric tear. Br J Surg 75: 786–788
Laurberg S, Swash M, Henry M M 1990 Effect of postanal repair on the progress of neurogenic damage to the pelvic floor. Br J Surg 77: 519–522
MacLeod J H 1987 Management of anal incontinence by biofeedback. Gastroenterology 93: 291–294

Mann C V and Hoffman C 1988 Complete rectal prolapse: the anatomical and functional results of treatment by an extended abdominal rectopexy. 75: 34–37

McHugh S M and Diamant N E 1987 Effect of age, gender and parity on anal canal pressures. Dig Dis Sci 32: 726–736

Miller R, Bartolo D C, Cervero F et al 1989 Differences in anal sensation in continent and incontinent patients with perineal descent. Int J Colon Dis 4: 45–49

Mortensen N, Smilgin Humphreys M 1991 The anal continence plug: a disposable device for patients with anorectal incontinence. Lancet 338: 295–297

Nelson R, Norton N, Cautley E 1994 Prevalence of faecal incontinence in Wisconsin households. Dis Colon Rectum 37: P9

Nielsen M B, Hauge C, Rasmussen O O et al 1992 Anal endosonographic findings in the follow–up of primarily sutured sphincteric ruptures. Br J Surg 79: 104–106

Parks A G 1975 Anorectal incontinence. J Royal Soc Med 68: 681–690

Read M, Read N W, Barber D C et al 1982 Effects of loperamide on anal sphincter function in patients complaining of chronic diarrhea with fecal incontinence and urgency. Dig Dis Sci 27: 807–814

Rogers J, Laurberg S, Misiewicz J J et al 1989 Anorectal physiology validated: a repeatable study of the motor and sensory tests of anorectal function. Br J Surg 76: 607–609

Seccia M, Menconi C, Balestri R et al 1994 Study protocols and functional results in 86 electrostimulated graciloplasties. Dis Colon Rectum 37: 897–904

Setti Carraro P, Kamm M A, Nicholls R J 1994 Long term results of postanal repair for neurogenic faecal incontinence. Br J Surg 81: 140–144

Shorvon P J, McHugh S, Diamant N E et al 1989 Defecography in normal volunteers: results and implications. Gut 30: 1737–1749

Snooks S J, Setchell M, Swash M et al 1984 Injury to innervation of pelvic floor sphincter musculature in childbirth. Lancet 2: 546–550

Snooks S J, Henry M M, Swash M 1985 Faecal incontinence due to external anal sphincter division in childbirth is associated with damage to the innervation of the pelvic floor musculature: a double pathology. Br J Obstet Gynaecol 92: 824–828

Snooks S J, Swash M, Mathers S E et al 1990 Effect of vaginal delivery on the pelvic floor: a 5-year follow–up. Br J Surg 77: 1358–1360

Sorensen S M, Bondesen H, Istre O et al 1988 Perineal rupture following vaginal delivery. Acta Obstet Gynecol Scand 67: 315–318

Sultan A H, Kamm M A, Hudson C N et al 1993a Anal-sphincter disruption during vaginal delivery. N Eng J Med 329: 1905–1911

Sultan A H, Kamm M A, Bartram C I et al 1993b Anal sphincter trauma during instrumental delivery. Int J Gynecol Obstet 43: 263–270

Sun W M, Read N W, Donnelly T C 1989 Impaired internal anal sphincter in a subgroup of patients with idiopathic fecal incontinence. Gastroenterology 97: 130–135

Williams N S, Patel J, George B D et al 1991 Development of an electrically stimulated neoanal sphincter. Lancet 338: 1166–1169

14

The management of vulval dystrophy

N. C. Gleeson

INTRODUCTION AND CLASSIFICATION

A plethora of terms has been applied to lesions characterized by shrinkage, whitening or reddening exclusive to the skin of the vulva. These include kraurosis, ichthyosis, lichen sclerosus, leukoplakia, leukokeratosis, neuro-dermatitis, Bowen's disease, hyperplastic vulvitis, Erythroplasia of Querat, and carcinoma simplex. Many of these terms have been used interchangeably as clinical and histological descriptions. The looseness of the terminology led to a wide range of treatments including radiotherapy and wide local excision for conditions of unproven malignant potential (Berkeley & Bonney 1909; Taussig 1929). The term chronic epithelial dystrophy was introduced by Jeffcoate & Woodcock (1961) to describe intractable vulval skin lesions of unknown aetiology. Gardner & Kaufman (1969) were the first to suggest a histopathological classification and their scheme was subsequently adapted by the International Society for the Study of Vulvar Disease (ISSVD) (Freidrich 1976).

The resulting ISSVD classification was:

> Hyperplastic Dystrophy
> with/without atypia
> Lichen sclerosus (hypoplastic dystrophy)
> Mixed dystrophy (lichen sclerosus with foci of epithelial hyperplasia)

This ISSVD classification is strictly histopathological and includes those vulval changes variously described in the past as leukoplakia, kraurosis, atrophic dystrophy, hyperplastic vulvitis, leukoplakic vulvitis and neuro-dermatitis. The dystrophic lesions may be diffuse or localized, thickened or thin, red or white in appearance. The histological features are described by Beilby & Ridley (1987).

As the term dystrophy suggests impaired nutrition or vascularization and there is no evidence of these processes in the aetiology of vulval dermatoses, the term 'dystrophy' was replaced by the term 'non neoplastic disorder of the vulva' in the subsequent reclassification by the ISSVD, shown in Table 14.1 (Ridley et al 1989). Squamous cell hyperplasia replaces hyperplastic

Table 14.1   Classification of Vulval Disorders (ISSVD 1989)

Non-neoplastic disorders of the vulva
Squamous cell hyperplasia (formerly hyperplastic dystrophy)
Lichen Sclerosus (formerly hypoplastic dystrophy)
Other dermatoses
Vulval Intraepithelial Neoplasia (VIN)
Squamous VIN
VIN I   Mild dysplasia
VIN II Moderate dysplasia
VIN II Severe dysplasia and carcinoma in situ
Non-squamous VIN
Paget's disease
Melanoma in situ

dystrophy and is used in those instances in which hyperplasia is not at-tributable to another cause. Dermatoses (e.g. psoriasis, lichen planus, con-dyloma acuminata) which demonstrate squamous hyperplasia and involve the vulva are excluded from the category of squamous hyperplasia and listed as other dermatoses. The finding of adjacent areas of squamous cell hy-perplasia with lichen sclerosus is regarded as part of the spectrum of lichen sclerosus and not evidence of another distinct dermatological condition. These cases are classified as lichen sclerosus with associated squamous cell hyperplasia. When intraepithelial neoplasia (VIN) occurs with dystrophy, both diagnoses should be reported e.g. squamous cell hyperplasia with VIN I, II or III.

MANAGEMENT OF VULVAL DYSTROPHY

The management of vulval dystrophy is guided by the type and severity of symptoms and the malignant potential of the lesion. The main symptoms of vulval dystrophy are chronic itching, burning, pain and superficial dyspareunia. The pruritus is often worst at night and can cause insomnia if severe. Vulval discharge or bleeding suggest the presence of infection or malignant ulceration. A thorough systemic review is essential as a vulval dermatosis may be part of a generalized dermatological condition (e.g. lichen planus, eczema, psoriasis, vitiligo, allergic dermatitis), a manifesta-tion of a multisystem disease (e.g. Behcet's, Crohn's disease, ulcerative colitis, sarcoidosis and amyloidosis), associated with autoimmune diseases (e.g. thyroid disease, pernicious anaemia, diabetes) or tumour (e.g. glucagonoma).

Examination of the patient must be general and inspection of the vulva, perianal area, vagina and cervix should be thorough. The diseased vulva can be extremely sensitive. The labia majora are parted gently. Continued out-ward and upward retraction of the anterior portion of the labia majora allows inspection of the clitoris and assessment of the mobility of the clitoral hood. Separation of the posterior half of the labia majora allows inspection of the introitus and further assessment of the mobility and thickness of the vulval tissues. The vulval lesions are best described in simple terms e.g. diffuse thinning and whitening of the skin; small raised red plaques. Terms such as leukoplakia should be avoided as they suggest a histological diagnosis which may be inaccurate. The preliminary examination should include speculum examination of the vagina and cervix (intraepithelial neoplastic lesions of the lower genital tract may be multifocal) and bimanual pelvic examination. If the vulva is very sensitive this part of the examination may need to be deferred.

Lichen sclerosus occurs most frequently in postmenopausal women and the classical appearance is of a white shrunken vulva with shiny papery skin on the vulva extending to encircle the anus in a figure-of-eight fashion, involutional adhesion of the labia minora to the labia majora, burying of the clitoris and shrinkage of the introitus. Up to 20% of patients with lichen sclerosus have extragenital lesions that present as small, ivory, shiny macules or papules that become atrophic and are usually asymptomatic. Bullous and haemorrhagic forms of these lesions have been described (Marren et al 1992a).

Extensive squamous hyperplastic dystrophy renders the vulval skin rubbery and redness may show through the white plaques. The appearance of a dystrophic vulva may change over time depending on the amount of moisture in the area and the extent of excoriation caused by scratching. Biopsy serves a dual purpose in diagnosing the type of skin lesion and excluding intra-epithelial or frank neoplasia. Recognition of possible sites of dysplasia (VIN) is difficult and colposcopic examination is of limited value (Soutter 1993). VIN is often raised above the surrounding skin and has a rough surface but the colour is variable depending on skin thickness and pigmentation. Acetic acid (5%) is applied for 3 minutes prior to examination. Colposcopic assessment is rendered difficult by the keratinisation of the skin and the size of the vulva and even early invasive cancer in VIN lesions can be missed (Chafe et al 1988). At best colposcopy will indicate suspicious areas from which biopsies should be taken. An alternative to colposcopy is a hand-held lens. The toluidine blue test is useful although limited by false negatives associated with hyperkeratosis and false positives due to excoriation (Cavanagh et al 1985). The test involves applying 1% aqueous toluidine blue to the vulva which is washed off with 1% acetic acid after 1 minute. Sky blue areas should be biopsied.

Biopsy of the vulva

Vulval biopsies can be performed in the gynaecologist's outpatient clinic using local anaesthetic and a Keyes punch biopsy instrument. The area should be cleansed with an antiseptic solution and local anaesthetic (1% lignocaine) is infiltrated under the skin with a 26 gauge needle. A 4 mm

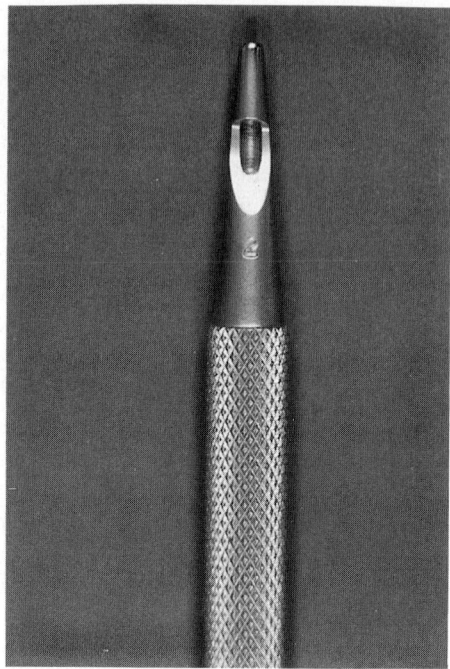

Fig. 14.1 Keyes punch biopsy.

Keyes punch biopsy instrument (Fig. 14.1) is then pressed against the skin and rotated clockwise and anticlockwise until a core of epidermis and dermis is obtained. Fine-toothed tissue forceps are used to lift the core of tissue which is freed at its tip with fine curved scissors. A silver nitrate impregnated cotton tip is applied to the biopsy site to achieve haemostasis. Biopsies of Lichen sclerosus (Fig. 14.2) and squamous, cell hyperflasia of the vulva (Fig. 14.3) are shown.

Treatment of vulval dystrophy

The preliminary treatment of vulval dystrophy is focused on the alleviation of symptoms, and further management is dictated by the risk of malignant progression and associated medical conditions. A dystrophic or scratched vulva can be aggravated by contact irritants such as deodorants, talcum powders, perfumed soaps and detergents, and changes in personal hygiene methods can improve symptoms. Marren et al (1992b) studied allergen patch testing in 135 patients with vulval pruritus and 63 had positive results. Of these 62% had positive results considered to be relevant to their clinical condition and more than half had multiple allergies. Cotton underwear and avoidance of synthetic tights reduce vulval moisture. Concomitant infections, e.g. candidiasis, should be treated. Urinary inconti-

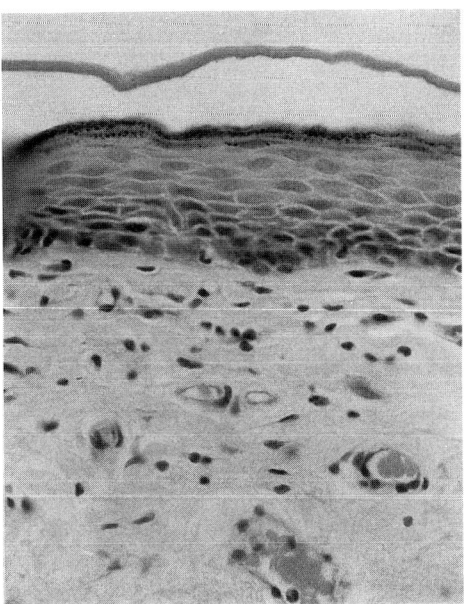

Fig. 14.2   Lichen sclerosus. Thinned squamous epithelium with effacement of the rete pegs and homogenization of the upper dermis, together with a sparse chronic inflammatory cell infiltrate.

nence should be corrected. Itching may be relieved by a topical corticosteroid such as 1% hydrocortisone aqueous cream or ointment. Other useful topical antipruritic agents include crotamiton and calamine. An oral antihistamine, e.g. chlorpheniramine 4 mg, at bedtime may help to break the itch-scratch cycle. Local anaesthetic gels such as 2% lignocaine give temporary relief of itching and can be kept in reserve for the intense bouts of itching such as those impairing sleep at night. In vulvodynia of unknown cause, the oral tricyclic drug, amitriptyline, in doses ranging from 10 to 60 mg/day is a useful adjunct to pain relief (McKay 1993). There are no data available on the use of such drugs in vulval dystrophy. For recalcitrant pruritus, Woodruff & Thompson (1972) described local injection of absolute alcohol into the superficial subcutaneous tissue of the vulva which provided relief of symptoms for up to 12 months, but the procedure carries a risk of sloughing of the tissues if the injection is either too superficial (epidermal) or too deep in the subcutaneous tissue.

   Steroid therapy.   Traditionally, topical corticosteroids are recommended to reverse the histological features of squamous hyperplasia. Lichen sclerosus has an atrophic histological appearance which makes treatment with an androgenic steroid seem more logical. Two percent testosterone propionate ointment applied twice daily initially for 3 to 6 weeks and then more sparingly (once or twice per week) is the standard recommended treatment for

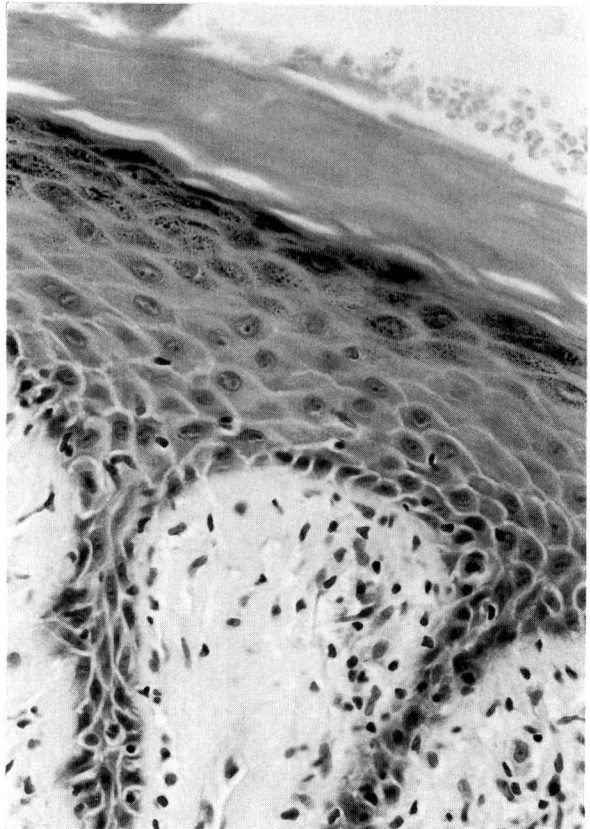

Fig. 14.3 Squamous cell hyperplasia of vulva. Hyperkeratosis, acanthosis with elongation of rete pegs and a chronic inflammatory cell infiltrate in the upper dermis.

lichen sclerosus. Excessive dosage of testosterone will result in virilization. Wright (1993) described subcutaneously implanted testosterone pellets which yielded extended remission of symptoms in lichen sclerosus. Mahmud et al (1992) reported symptomatic improvement and reduction in lesion size in 80% of lichen sclerosus and 89% of squamous hyperplasia patients treated with testosterone and corticosteroid respectively, in a small series. Oestrogen may have little or no direct effect on the epidermis but improves the vascularity of the underlying dermis. Oestrogen replacement therapy should be considered in postmenopausal women with vulval dystrophy.

Controlled studies of clobetasol. There are few controlled or randomized studies on the treatment of vulval dystrophy. Bracco et al (1993) randomized 79 patients with histologically proven lichen sclerosus to one of four treatment modalities in an unblinded fashion: clobetasol propionate 0.05%, testosterone in petroleum 2%, progesterone in petroleum 2% and a placebo. The symptoms, gross appearance and histology were scored and repeated after 3 months of treatment. Only the clobetasol group improved significantly. Dalziel et al (1993) performed an open study on twice daily applications of clobetasol propionate 0.05% (Dermovate, Glaxo, UK) in 12 patients and followed their progress for 39 months. They reported symptomatic and histological improvement and the only long-term side effect was background erythema. Most patients subsequently required only less potent corticosteroids to control their symptoms. Carli et al (1994) described activation of the epidermal antigen-presenting cells and lymphoid cells with an increase in the epidermal Langerhan's cells (CD1a+ cells), which suggests involvement of the skin's immune system in the pathogenesis of lichen sclerosus. Conventional topical 2% testosterone failed to modify these immunohistological features, but 0.05% clobetasol down-regulated the skin's immune system activation profile in 20 patients with vulval lichen sclerosus. Therefore, topical clobetasol emerges as a drug that is effective in the control of symptoms and reverses histological and immunohistological changes in vulval lichen sclerosus.

Treatment with retinoids.   Promising results are also emerging from treatment of vulval lichen sclerosus with oral retinoids. These vitamin A analogues have been used for generalized dermatological conditions for over a decade. Bousema et al (1994) studied the efficacy of acitretin (20–30 mg/day) for 16 weeks in a randomized, double-blind, placebo-controlled trial in 78 patients. A satisfactory response was obtained in 64% of acitretin-treated patients compared to 25% given placebo. The retinoids are teratogenic and because of their highly lipophilic nature, can be stored in adipose tissue for up to 2 years after discontinuation of therapy. Fortunately, the majority of vulval dystrophy occurs in postmenopausal women. Younger women need to be counselled about the teratogenic risk and the need for effective contraception. Other adverse reactions to retinoids include skin dryness and peeling, eye irritation, temporary hair loss, myalgia and pseudoporphyria. When vulval dystrophy occurs in association with human papilloma virus infection, intralesional injection of interferon-alpha-2b has been described with relief of chronic vulval discomfort and limited reversal of the histological changes (Larsen et al 1993, Sonnendecker et al 1993). The management of other dermatoses associated with a general dermatological condition should be undertaken by a dermatologist.

Surgical treatment

Simple vulvectomy for chronic vulval dystrophy was previously advocated to prevent progression to invasive cancer. However, dystrophy often reappeared in the transposed skin over the excised area. Histologically proven dystrophy is no longer an indication for such aggressive surgery. Meyrich-Thomas et al (1988) estimated that 4% of women with lichen sclerosus develop invasive cancer. There are certainly case reports of invasive cancer developing in lichen sclerosus (Hofman & Megahed 1994) and co-existence of VIN and invasive cancer with lichen sclerosus has been described by many authors (Stening & Elliott 1959; Leibowitch et al 1990; Micheletti et al 1994; Ansink et al 1994). Currently, asymptomatic patients with vulval dystrophy are not always treated. We do not yet know if the reversal of the histological and immunohistological features of lichen sclerosus by clobetasol also reduces the risk of malignant progression. Squamous hyperplasia and mixed dystrophy are more likely to be associated with atypia and invasive cancer (Elliott 1988). The treatment of VIN has become more conservative with recognition that spontaneous regression can occur and the suggestion that progression to invasive disease may be less likely in younger women (Barbero et al 1993), but Jones & Rowan (1994) refute the latter suggestion and recommend early treatment of VIN III based on their findings in a retrospective series of 113 patients. While dystrophy is usually a disease of the postmenopausal years, VIN occurs more frequently in the 20- to 40-year-old age group of women and any surgical procedure on the vulva has to be viewed in the context of cosmetic and functional impairment. The treatment modalities include wide local excision, vulvectomy, laser, cautery and chemotherapy. The ablative techniques (laser and cautery) are limited in their value by not providing a histological specimen and allowing residual disease to persist in the skin appendages. Topical chemotherapy can cause extensive excoriation and ulceration. Excisional biopsies for Paget's disease should include the subcutaneous tissue so that underlying adenocarcinoma can be excluded, but need not include a wide margin of normal skin as recurrence rates are about 12% regardless of the extent of histological involvement (Freidrich 1981). The risk of recurrence is high with any intraepithelial neoplasia of the vulva.

Follow-up

Long-term surveillance of patients with vulval dystrophy is recommended. The overall risk of malignant progression may be small but surgical cure rates for early invasive cancer are excellent and early diagnosis allows use of a modified approach to radical vulvectomy. Vulval self-examination using a mirror in a squatting or sitting position can be taught and patients should be encouraged to report any worrying changes. Biopsies should be performed if any suspicious lesions such as ulcers appear. Regular review of a dystrophic vulva is also recommended for reassessment of the patients symptoms and to offer psychological support in a condition that can seriously impair the quality of a woman's life.

KEY POINTS FOR CLINICAL PRACTICE

1. Patients suspected of having vulval dystrophy/non-neoplastic vulval epithelial disorder should have the diagnosis confirmed histologically.

2. Vulval biopsy can be performed in the gynaecologist's outpatient clinic.

3. Old terminology is now obsolete. Two histological types are specific to the vulva – lichen sclerosus and squamous hyperplasia and these may co-exist.

4. Traditionally, treatment was tailored to the histological type. Lichen sclerosus (hypoplastic dystrophy) was treated with topical testosterone. Squamous hyperplasia (hyperplastic dystrophy) was treated with topical corticosteroids. Long-term use of testosterone can cause virilization. Long-term use of corticosteroids can cause excessive atrophy. More recently, a potent topical corticosteroid (clobetasol) has been shown to be effective in lichen sclerosus.

5. Vulval dystrophy associated with vulval intraepithelial neoplasia (VIN) should be managed as VIN.

6. Long-term follow-up is required because of the small risk of malignant progression and the need to review symptoms and provide psychological support.

REFERENCES

Ansink A C, Krul M R, De Weger R A et al 1994 Human papillomavirus, lichen sclerosus, and squamous cell carcinoma of the vulva: detection and prognostic significance. Gynecol Oncol 52: 180–184

Barbero M, Micheletti L, Preti M et al 1993 Biological behavior of vulvar intraepithelial neoplasms. Histological and clinical presentation. J Reprod Med 38: 108–112

Beilby J O W, Ridley C M 1987 The pathology of the vulva. In: Fox H (ed) Haines and Taylor Obstetrical and Gynaecological Pathology, 3rd edition. Churchill Livingstone, Edinburgh, pp 64–145

Berkeley C, Bonney V 1909 Leukoplakic vulvitis and its relation to kraurosis vulvae and carcinoma vulvae. Proc Royal Soc Med 3 (2): 29–51

Bousema M T, Romppanen U, Geiger J M et al 1994 Acitretin in the treatment of severe lichen sclerosus et atrophicus of the vulva: a double-blind, placebo-controlled study. J Am Acad Dermatol 30: 225–231

Bracco G L, Carli P, Sonni L et al 1993 Clinical and histological effects of topical treatments of vulval lichen sclerosis: A critical evaluation. J Reprod Med 38: 37–42

Carli P, Bracco G, Taddei G et al 1994 Vulvar lichen sclerosus. Immunohistological evaluation before and after therapy. J Reprod Med 39: 110–114

Cavanagh D, Ruffolo E H, Marsden D E 1985 Cancer of the Vulva. In: Cavanagh D (ed) Gynecologic Cancer. A clinicopathological approach. Appleton-Century-Crofts, Connecticut, pp 1–40

Chafe W, Richards A, Morgan L, Wilkinson E 1988 Unrecognised invasive carcinoma in vulvar intraepithelial neoplasia (VIN). Gynecol Oncol 31: 154–165

Dalziel K L, Wojnarowska F 1993 Long term control of vulval lichen sclerosus after treatment with a potent topical steroid cream. J Reprod Med 38: 25–27

Elliott P 1988 Vulvar cancer after treatment of microinvasive lesions. J Reprod Med 33: 717 (Abstr.)

Freidrich E G 1976 New nomenclature for vulvar disease. Report of the Committee on terminology. Obstet Gynecol 47: 122–124

Freidrich E G 1981 Intraepithelial neoplasia of the vulva. In: Coppleson M (ed) Gynecologic Oncology: Fundamental Principles and Clinical Practice. Churchill, New York, p 303

Gardner H L, Kaufman R H 1969. Benign diseases of the vulva and vagina. Mosby C V (ed), St. Louis, Missoon

Hofman U, Megahed M 1994 Spinocellular cancer in lichen sclerosus et atrophicus of the vulva. Hautarzt 45: 104–107

Jeffcoate T N A, Woodcock A S 1961 Premalignant conditions of the vulva, with particular reference to chronic epithelial dystrophies. Br Med J ii: 127–134

Jones R W, Rowan D M 1994 Vulvar intraepithelial neoplasia III: A clinical study of the outcome of 113 cases with relation to the later development of invasive vulvar carcinoma. Obstet Gynecol 84: 741–745

Larsen J, Peters K, Petersen C S et al 1993 Interferon alpha-2b treatment of symptomatic chronic vulvodynia associated with koilocytosis. Acta Dermatol Venereol 73: 385–387

Leibowitch M, Neill S, Pelisse M, Moyal-Barracco M 1990 The epithelial changes associated with squamous cell carcinoma of the vulva. A review of the clinical histological and viral findings in 78 women. Br J Obstet Gynaecol 97: 1135–1139

Mahmud M, Murakami T, Gyotoku Y, Nakazima H, Ishimuru T, Yamabe T 1992 Vulvar dystrophy: a clinical follow-up. Asia Oceania Journal of Obstetrics & Gynaecology 18: 231–238

Marren P, DeBecker D, Millard P, Wojnarowska F 1992a Bullous and haemorrhagic lichen sclerosus with scalp involvement. Clin Experiment Dermatol 17: 354–356

Marren P, Wojnarowska F, Powell S 1992b Allergic contact dermatitis and vulvar dermatoses. Br J Dermatol 126: 52–56

Meyrick-Thomas R H, Ridley C M, McGibbon D H, Black M M 1988 Lichen Sclerosus and autoimmunity–a study of 350 women. Br J Dermatol 118: 41–46

Micheletti L, Barbero M, Preti M et al 1994 Vulvar intraepithelial neoplasia of low grade: a challenging diagnosis. Eur J Gynaecol Oncol 15: 70–74

McKay M 1993 Dysesthetic ('essential') vulvodynia: Treatment with Amitriptyline. J Reprod Med 38: 9–13

Ridley C M, Frankman O, Jones I S C et al 1989 New nomenclature in vulvar disease: International society for the study of vulvar disease. Hum Pathol 20: 495–496

Sonnendecker E W, Sonnendecker H E, Wright C A, Simon G B 1993 Recalcitrant vulvodynia. A clinicopathological study. S Afr Med J 83: 730–733

Souter P 1993 Colposcopy of the vulva. In: Souter (ed) A Practical Guide to Colposcopy. Oxford University Press, Oxford, pp 161–186

Stening M, Elliott P M 1959 Primary carcinoma of the vulva with special reference to leukoplakia. J Obstet Gynaecol British Empire 66: 897–904

Taussig F J 1929 Leukoplakic vulvitis and cancer of the vulva (etiology, histopathology, treatment, five-year results). Am J Obstet Gynecol 18: 472–503

Wright A J 1993 Testosterone pellet implant therapy for lichen sclerosus. Mod Med 90: 711–713

Woodruff J D, Thompson B 1972 Local injection in the treatment of vulvar pruritus. Obstet Gynecol 40: 18–22

Index